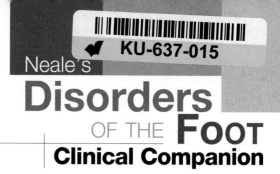

KU-637-015

Neale's

Disorders
OF THE FOOT
Clinical Companion

Commissioning Editor: *Robert Edwards/Sarena Wolfaard*
Development Editor: *Nicola Lally*
Project Manager: *Nayagi Athmanathan*
Designer/Design Direction: *Charles Gray*
Illustration Manager: *Gillian Richards*
Illustrator: *Jane Fallows*

Neale's

Disorders

OF THE FOOT
Clinical Companion

Paul Frowen MPhil, FCHS, FCPodMed, DPodM
Head of Wales Centre for Podiatric Studies, Principal Lecturer, Podiatry, University of Wales Institute, Cardiff, UK

Maureen O'Donnell BSc(Hons), FChS, FPodMed, DPod M, Dip Ed
Podiatrist; Former Programme Leader, Senior Lecturer, Division of Podiatric Medicine and Surgery, Glasgow Caledonian University, UK

Donald L Lorimer B Ed (Hons), FCPodMed, MChS, DPod M
Podiatrist, Former Head of School, Durham School of Podiatric Medicine; Past Chairman of Council The Society of Chiropodists and Podiatrists; Former Co-ordinator Joint Quality Assurance Committee of the Society of Chiropodists and Podiatrists/Health Professions Council; Health Professions Council Partner, UK

Gordon Burrow DPodM, BA, AdvDipEd, FChS, MPhil, FCPodMed, MSc, CMIOSH, FHEA
Podiatrist, Senior Lecturer, Department of Diagnostic Imaging, Operating Department Practice, Podiatry and Radiotherapy, School of Health, Glasgow Caledonian University, Glasgow, UK

Foreword by
Val Brewster

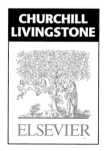

CHURCHILL LIVINGSTONE

ELSEVIER

Edinburgh   London   New York   Oxford   Philadelphia   St Louis   Sydney   Toronto   2010

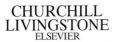

CHURCHILL
LIVINGSTONE
ELSEVIER

ISBN 978-0-7020-3171-7

British Library Cataloguing in Publication Data
A catalogue record for this book is available from the British Library

Library of Congress Cataloging in Publication Data
A catalog record for this book is available from the Library of Congress

Notices
Knowledge and best practice in this field are constantly changing. As new research and experience broaden our understanding, changes in research methods, professional practices, or medical treatment may become necessary.

Practitioners and researchers must always rely on their own experience and knowledge in evaluating and using any information, methods, compounds, or experiments described herein. In using such information or methods they should be mindful of their own safety and the safety of others, including parties for whom they have a professional responsibility.

With respect to any drug or pharmaceutical products identified, readers are advised to check the most current information provided (i) on procedures featured or (ii) by the manufacturer of each product to be administered, to verify the recommended dose or formula, the method and duration of administration, and contraindications. It is the responsibility of practitioners, relying on their own experience and knowledge of their patients, to make diagnoses, to determine dosages and the best treatment for each individual patient, and to take all appropriate safety precautions.

To the fullest extent of the law, neither the Publisher nor the authors, contributors, or editors, assume any liability for any injury and/or damage to persons or property as a matter of products liability, negligence or otherwise, or from any use or operation of any methods, products, instructions, or ideas contained in the material herein.

Printed in China

Contents

Foreword

In 1981 when my grandfather, Donald Neale, completed the 1st edition of his book 'Common Foot Disorders' he would never have imagined that the book would become the academic heavyweight that the 8th edition is today. His work always played a part in my life, from my visits to him at the Edinburgh Foot Clinic (usually for treatment of my verrucae) to my fascination with the gruesome photographs that were always on his desk. My grandfather was so proud of me when I started nursing but I wish he had known that I was to have a career change and follow in his footsteps shortly after his death in 1997. His dedication to his family and the profession was absolute and this and his hard work was a major contributor to the progression of the profession.

The original title of 'Common Foot Disorders' is no longer suitable for this book which has developed to meet the increased scope of practice of the podiatrist, the ever evolving curriculum for students and the CPD requirements for practitioners. A vast range of foot disorders and systemic related pathologies including, rheumatology, vascular disorders, dermatology and diabetes are covered in detail. Whilst the text is thorough it is enhanced by explicit diagrams, tables and photographs. Some of the foot conditions and related disorders are not necessarily seen in everyday clinical practice but recognition, diagnosis, referral and management is a requirement for today's clinicians and this book meets these needs. A Clinical Companion and an interactive Web Base is now available with the 8th edition.

The 8th edition is an invaluable source of references and updated material for practitioners and other health care professionals. It continues to focus on, and deliver, updated learning material for students and comprehensively covers topics required for their clinical experience, examinations and assessments. The web pages include video clips and self assessment multiple-choice questions all of which are clinically relevant to students and practitioners. Several chapters have been altered, amalgamated or streamlined to reflect current practice. Leprosy and Tropical Diseases have been combined, Musculoskeletal Disorders updated and there is a new slant on the chapter dealing with the podiatric problems of the elderly patient. Therapeutic footwear is now an addition within the footwear chapter and the medical emergencies chapter is very appropriate to current podiatric practice.

The addition of the clinical companion and web based interactive material is a huge step forward. The clinical companion is based on the main book and is an excellent resource for a quick reference clinical tool or revision, with concise information which is easy to access and is very relevant to the clinical situation. To have such a variety of learning tools is excellent; it helps to consolidate information in a memorable and interesting way.

The 8th edition continues to extend the work started by my grandfather 30 years ago. It clearly reflects the great strides which have been made in the profession since the first edition. I am certain that all podiatry practitioners will find this an invaluable and informative book.

Valerie Brewster
Private Practitioner
Bearsden Foot Clinic

Preface

The first edition of Neales's Disorders of the foot was produced by Donald Neale in 1981, with the intention of developing a book that incorporated the many diverse bodies of medical and biological knowledge that are essential components of the profession of podiatry. Prior to this most of the literature that had been specifically developed for the profession had been written in the years preceding World War 2 and whilst revised to reflect changes in practice were very much embedded in the fourth decade of the twentieth century.

Neale's Disorders of the foot, has incrementally evolved since the first edition which represented UK podiatric practice in the late 1970s. Podiatric practice and education has developed significantly within the past 30 years both in respect of scope of practice and educational changes that were required to support practice. All approved programmes of Podiatry in the UK are now normally at honours degree level or above. Increasing numbers of podiatrist now have higher degrees and this has contributed to the breadth of the evidence base upon which best practice is founded.

The seven previous editions of the text have endeavoured to be a focus for the knowledge base of the profession whilst giving emphasis to the place it holds within the wider field of patient care. Similarly the eighth edition strives to continue this function and many chapters have been revised or rewritten and a number of new contributors have provided a fresh approach to some of the content.

The layout and content of chapters in the eighth edition followed much thought and there have been a number of changes which place some elements in more logically clinically related locations and where possible duplication of information has been minimised. The need for the text to provide for the needs of both the student podiatrist and the practitioner has been at the forefront of our deliberations and it is hoped that this edition continues to provide a ready reference from assessment to diagnosis and management.

Within our consideration of the content and focus of the eighth edition, the need to develop a clinical companion that provided a digest of the main text became apparent. We hope that this new text will be a useful addition which will serve as a source of information within clinical settings and that it like the main text will grow and develop in each new edition to reflect the changes that will inevitably occur within the profession.

Paul Frowen
2010

Acknowledgements

The editors are indebted and grateful to the following authors for their comments and amendments upon the chapters we have abridged for the companion:

Asra Ahmad, James A Black, Jacqueline Saxe Buchman, Robert Campbell, Bev Durrant, Michael E Edmonds, Brian M. Ellis, Jeffrey Evans, J Douglas Forrest, Dr Krishna Goel, Robert James Hardie, Farina Hashmi, Phillip Helliwell, Margaret Johnson, Tom Lucke, Peter Madigan, Ian Mathieson, Jonathan McGhie, Alistair McInnes, Janet McInnes, Jean Mooney, Colin Munro, Anthony Redmond, David T Roberts, Michael Graham Serpell, Christine M Skinner, Kate Springett, John Thomson, Wendy Tyrrell, Gordon F Watt, Anne Whinfield.

We hope that we have reflected their views within this distillation of their work and that it serves as a supportive text in clinical practice.

We also would like to express our gratitude Mrs Valerie Brewster (Donald Neale's Granddaughter) who was able to provide the foreword. Her personal references provided a touching insight into the man originally responsible for Neale's Disorders of the foot.

Last but not least, we are also most appreciative of the help and assistance provided by Ms Nicola Lally, Mr Robert Edwards, Ms Nayagi Athmanathan and Sarena Wolfaard in the development and production of this edition.

Chapter 1

Examination and diagnosis in clinical management

Elements of any history will include the following as shown in Fig 1.1.

INTRODUCTORY INFORMATION

Introductory information includes date of the history, identifying data or demographics (age, sex, race, place of birth, marital status, occupation, religion), source of referral (if any), source and reliability of the history and leads onto the chief complaints.

CHIEF COMPLAINTS – SOLICITING CONTRIBUTION

The main focus of the history is the prime reason why the patient has presented to the practitioner. A detailed and thorough investigation into the current concern is vital comprising two essential but combined parts:

- first, the patient's account of the symptoms (ensure that it is the patient's and not the view of another, for example a carer or parent), that is the subjective symptoms
- secondly, the objective signs – those detected by the skill of the practitioner. The main aim is to obtain a comprehensive, succinct account from the patient's perspective of the presenting symptom(s).

PAST MEDICAL HISTORY

Includes the general state of health, childhood illnesses (remember age of patient and country of birth), adult illnesses, psychiatric illness, accidents and injuries, operations and hospitalisations. This helps gauge the patient overall, and how they view health and disease.

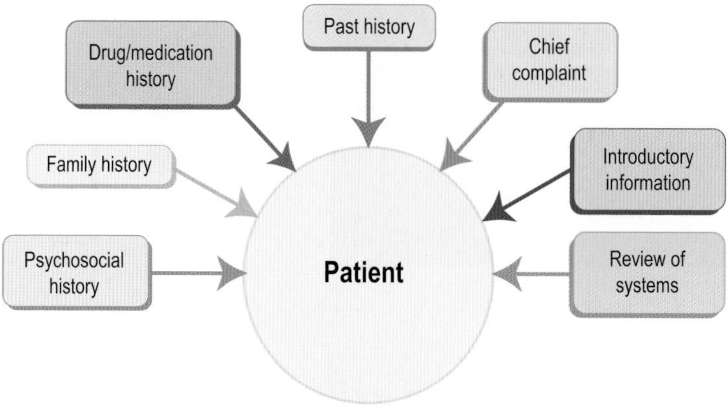

Figure 1.1 Elements of a history.

DRUG/MEDICATION HISTORY

It is advisable to request this information before the first appointment by advising the patient to present with a list of current medication (prescribed and over-the-counter medicine) with the dosage of the medicine.

The drug history may give an indication of current illness. It is important to include home remedies, vitamin/mineral supplements, borrowed medicines as well as the prescription-only medicines (POM) and over-the-counter (OTC) variety.

SOCIAL HISTORY

It is important to establish how the disease or complaint and patient interact at a functional level. Try to establish what the patient's normal daily activities are and how their complaint has affected them.

FAMILY HISTORY

Information about the health and age of other members of the family can be constructive, particularly where there may be a genetic link to disorders.

REVIEW OF SYSTEMS

- *General* – identify factors such as height, weight, recent weight changes, fatigue or fever.
- *Skin* – look for rashes, lumps, sores, itching, dryness, colour changes, or changes in hair or nails. These may well indicate systemic conditions, such as diabetes, rheumatoid disease.
- *Respiratory* – signs of asthma, bronchitis, emphysema or past history of tuberculosis.

- *Cardiac* – heart trouble, high blood pressure, rheumatic fever, heart murmurs, chest pain, palpitations and results of any heart tests.
- *Urinary* – frequency of urination, polyuria, nocturia or burning pain on urination.
- *Endocrine* – thyroid trouble, heat or cold intolerance, excessive sweating, or excessive hunger or thirst.
- *Haematological* – anaemia, easy bruising or bleeding, past transfusions and possible reactions.
- *Neurological* – fainting, blackouts, seizures, weakness, paralysis, numbness, tingling, tremor or involuntary movements.
- *Peripheral vascular* – intermittent claudication, leg cramps or varicose veins.

ATTRIBUTES OF SYMPTOMS

The principal symptoms should be described using seven basic attributes:

- location
- quality
- quantity or severity
- timing (onset, duration, frequency)
- setting
- factors which aggravate or relieve
- associated manifestations.

PHYSICAL EXAMINATION Fig 1.2

The general survey should give an overall impression of the patient's general attributes, but these may well vary according to socioeconomic status, nutrition, genetic makeup, early illness, gender and the country and era of birth. The overview should encompass areas such as:

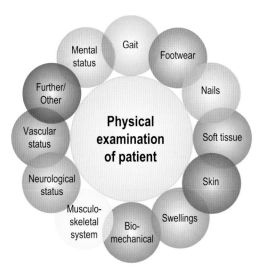

Figure 1.2 Physical examination of patient.

- apparent state of health – robust, acutely or chronically ill, frail
- signs of distress – laboured breathing, wincing, limping, sweatiness, trembling
- skin colour – pallor, cyanosis, jaundice, rashes, and bruises
- height and build – tall, short, muscular, disproportionate, symmetrical, e.g. Turner's syndrome (child may be short stature)
- weight by appearance or measurement – emaciated, slender, plump, fat, obese, although this may remain controversial as to appropriate weight
- posture, motor ability and gait – posture, which aids breathing, or pain, ataxia, limp, and paralysis – does the patient walk easily, confidently, balanced?
- dress, grooming, and personal hygiene – excessive clothes of hypothyroidism, long sleeves to cover rashes, or needle marks. Is the patient wearing unusual jewellery such as copper bands which might indicate arthritis? Is personal hygiene reflective of the patient's mood, personality, lifestyle, occupation and socio-economic grouping?
- facial expressions – observe these throughout the encounter, during the physical examination – immobile face of Parkinsonism, grimace when certain areas touched
- odour of body or breath – breath odour of alcohol, acetone (diabetes).

Mental status

The patient's mental status throughout the consultation should be observed, indicating the appropriateness of behaviour, the ability of the patient to comply with any management plan suggested.

Skin (see also Chapter 2)

Look and observe, touch and palpate skin over the foot and lower limb and seek answers to the following areas:

- texture: course, fine, dull or shiny, smooth or rough
- colour: cyanosis, jaundice, changes in melanin, pallor, erythema, pigmentation, gangrene
- temperature: cool, warm, distinctly hot, normal temperature gradient
- humidity: moist, dry, oily, areas of maceration, dryness associated with hypothyroidism, oiliness in acne
- elasticity: mobility; ease with which a fold of skin can be moved; decreased in oedema
- hyperkeratosis: corns and callus formation, sites, texture and quality
- hair: presence, absence, quantity, thickness, distribution, texture
- integrity: fissures (heel or interdigital clefts especially), ulcers, abrasions
- dermatoses: eczema, psoriasis
- surgical interventions: scars, infections.

Nails (see also Chapter 3)

Inspect and palpate these, identifying:

- the structure – ridged, cracked, thickened
- extent – overgrown, onychogryphotic, stunted, ingrowing, chewed, picked

- colour – cyanosis, pallor
- shape – club, excessive curvature
- subungual abnormality – swelling, pigmentation
- lesions – paronychia, onycholysis.

Swellings

Palpate and inspect any swellings and note:

- tenderness – local or radiating
- consistency – hard, firm, soft, fluctuant
- adherence to underlying structures – to skin, underlying soft tissues, to bone
- transillumination – does swelling transilluminate to light?
- temperature.

Musculoskeletal system (see also Chapter 8)

- Ease and range of motion – assess for limitation in movement, but also unusual increase in mobility of the joint which might lead to instability. Range of motion varies between individuals and decreases with age
- Signs of inflammation and swelling in or around the joint
- Condition of the surrounding tissues – should include matters such as muscle atrophy, subcutaneous nodules and skin changes
- Crepitus or crepitation, which is palpable
- Any musculoskeletal deformities, including abnormal curvatures of the spine should be assessed.

Footwear (see also Chapter 18)

Footwear gives a variety of clues as to diagnosis; therefore, it should also be examined during the patient's first visit. Footwear should initially be checked for size, shape, style, suitability for foot and occupation and indications of (abnormal) wear marks.

Vascular assessment (see also Chapter 5)

- Arterial:
  - pulses – DP, PT, AT
  - colour
  - temperature
  - skin
  - nails
  - hair
  - capillary refill time
  - pain/intermittent claudication
- Venous:
  - swelling
  - oedema
  - varicosity
  - haemosiderin deposits
  - cramping
- Lymphatic system:
  - swelling.

NEUROLOGICAL ASSESSMENT (see also Chapter 6)

Motor system

The main aim in examining the motor system is to:

- identify any lesions
- ascertain whether the lesion is an *upper motor neurone* (UMN) or a *lower motor neurone* (LMN) lesion
- locate the anatomical site
- consider the differential diagnosis of lesions at that site.

  The examination should follow a routine:

- inspection
- palpation
- assessment of motor tone
- assessment of power
- assessment of reflexes
- assessment of co-ordination
- assessment of gait.

  (Not necessarily in that order.)

Sensory investigations

Light touch

Dab a cotton wool ball onto the skin lightly. If an area of sensory diminution is suggested attempt to map this out. Start from the area of decreased sensation to an area of normal sensation.

Pin prick

As pain and temperature run in the same tract (spinothalamic) it is only necessary to perform one of the tests rather than both, unless some concern or questions remain having performed one.

Vibration

Sensations of the posterior column are position and vibration sensation.

Pressure

Semmes-Weinstein monofilaments

Used as a predictor of foot ulceration, especially in diabetes. These filaments are tested on various areas of the foot as described in Fig 1.3.

> **For more information see**
> **Neale's Disorders of the Foot 8E**   *page 12*

Gait

Analysis of gait is rudimentary and should be carried out routinely when first seeing the patient.

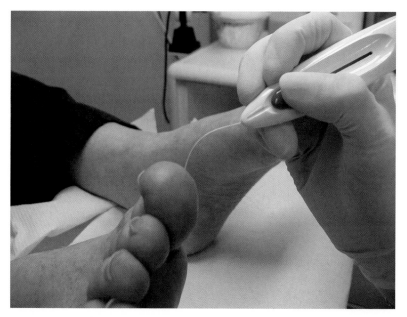

Figure 1.3 Use of the Semmes-Weinstein mono-filament to test for pressure – a 10 mg filament.

It is best to observe the gait when the patient is unaware of the observation. Gait analysis can either be by simple observation or by various measuring devices and mechanical methods.

Video recording enables the more subtle changes or patterns to be viewed and repeated but this is not always possible.

Static evaluation

The *plantarscope* shows how the plantar surface of tissues blanches on loading. This consists of a platform with a safety glass platform, over an angled mirror, allowing a view of the plantar surface of the foot. The *podometer* is more elaborate and combines measurements of foot size and calcaneal deviation with the reflected image. The *pedobaroscope* is an internally lit sheet of glass with a plastic or paper card interface. The person stands on the interface and reflected light is produced as a grey-scale image. This is stored or a hard copy produced for analysis.

Dynamic evaluation

Various devices are now available. The simplest device is possibly a sheet of black paper. The feet are dusted with chalk and the patient then walks the length of the sheet or roll of black paper. Inkless paper systems are also available, such as Podotracks and other systems.

More sophisticated systems such as the Musgrave, Kistler forceplate, etc. are available.

Other soft tissues

Some clinical signs should be given greater importance than others. The most important of all clinical signs is that of the inflammatory process, classically described as:

- rubor (redness)
- calor (warmth)
- dolor (pain)
- tumor (swelling)
- loss of function is another classic sign of the inflammatory process. Again, accurate recording of the features will enhance clinical practice.

The record card should indicate:

- if acute, chronic or subacute
- if infected, whether localised, and if suppurating or resolving
- if infected and spreading, what other tissues are involved – cellulitis, lymphadenitis, lymphangitis
- if pus is produced, what the colour and texture and fluidity is like – this will enable comparison between streptococcal and staphylococcal infections.

Any acute or subacute inflammatory lesion requires priority over a deformity, while that of a spreading infection requires immediate referral for further investigation and management.

BIOMECHANICAL EXAMINATION
(see also Chapter 14)

Assessment of the joint complexes of the foot and ankle and their relationships to the lower extremity and spinal column are vital to any diagnosis of foot problems of a structural or functional nature.

Motion of any joints within their normal range should be pain-free and unrestricted. The features of pain, crepitus, restricted movement or excessive motion may suggest a joint pathology.

Deformity affecting either of the osseous components of the joint or tenderness affecting the surrounding structures on palpation may also indicate pathology.

The various complexes of the foot and ankle should be assessed and examined individually.

FURTHER INVESTIGATIONS

Some simple further tests may be initiated by podiatrists to enable a more reliable diagnosis and management plan to be conducted. These require taking of samples of various constituent parts of the body and would require communication to the patient as to why these samples were needed and what was expected to be obtained from them.

APPLYING CRITICAL THINKING TO
THE INFORMATION GATHERED

Data gathered through the above processes may be either partial or complete, but such data now require analysis. This is achieved using the following steps:

- identify the abnormal findings that include the symptoms, physical signs and any available laboratory test findings.
- cluster or organise these findings into a logical group or groups.

- localise the findings anatomically – the clinician may have to settle for a body region (i.e. the foot) or for a system (musculoskeletal) or may be able to define the exact nature and location (spring ligament).
- interpret the findings in terms of the probable process:
  - *pathological* – abnormality in body structure – processes such as inflammatory, traumatic, toxic, vascular
  - *pathophysiological* – abnormality in function
  - *psychopathological* – disorder of mood or thinking.
- attempt to interpret these findings and cluster them to form a hypothesis or probable diagnosis.
- eliminate a hypothesis that fails to explain the findings.
- weigh the probability of a different hypothesis or diagnosis according to:
  - the match with the findings
  - statistical probability of a given disease in a patient of this age, sex, race, habits, lifestyle, locality and other variables
  - the timing of the patient's illness
- test the diagnosis. This may require further history, additional physical examination or laboratory tests. The clinician may require consultation with, or referral to, other specialists.
- establish a working definition of the problem.

CREATING THE RECORD

The patient's record is not just a record of what was done to the patient by the chiropodist/practitioner – it is legal documentation of the consultation process.

The record should be:

- accurate
- clear
- well organised
- up-to-date
- legible.

It should emphasise the important features and omit the irrelevant.

Abbreviations and symbols used should be those commonly used and understood; diagrams add greatly to the clarity of records where appropriate and measurements should be in centimetres and not obtuse inaccurate schemes of measurement such as pea-sized!

SOAPE system is one such recording method, ensuring accuracy and completeness of data for each consultation.

S = symptoms described by the patient
O = objective signs observed by practitioner
A = action taken that day
P = plan of management for patient as agreed between the two parties
E = evaluation of previous treatment given, and thus gives a synopsis of how the management plan is progressing.

Chapter | 2 |

The skin and nail disorders in podiatry

Clinical observation of the skin and nails is an important aspect of the process of assessment and diagnosis of the patient. There are many indicators provided by these easily observed structures that can very quickly point the way to an accurate diagnosis.

Examination can provide diagnostic indicators of various systemic disorders, examples of which are pruritus (itchiness) with chronic liver disease or bullae (blisters) with an adverse drug reaction. It also provides an indication of the quality of peripheral tissues both superficial and deep. The skin will show physical changes, for example the microcirculation in diabetes, that are also likely to be occurring in the deeper tissues not visible to the clinician.

It should be noted that changes with age are normal.

STRUCTURE AND FUNCTION OF THE SKIN

The skin is the largest of the body's organs and has a number of roles which includes protection, interaction with the environment and homeostasis.

The three main components of the skin are the epidermis, the dermoepidermal junction (DEJ, basement membrane) and the dermis, which is further divided into layers.

ACUTE INFLAMMATION

Human tissues respond to trauma by a complex series of events that have yet to be fully understood. This trauma may be mechanical, thermal, photo, chemical, or brought about through allergic or autoimmune events.

Damaged tissues will release chemical messengers which start the inflammatory process. Sequential phases of proliferation, maturation and repair of the damaged tissue follow inflammation, in health. Table 2.1

Table 2.1 Some chemical/inflammatory mediators which cause the features of inflammation

Histamine Kinins Prostaglandins Leucotrienes	From a variety of sources, including mast cells, macrophages, platelets
Complement component Plasma Cytokines	Have differing functions according to predominance and sequence of release, so different types of inflammatory responses occur

The classic and clinical features of inflammation are redness (rubor), heat (calor), swelling (tumor) and pain (dolor); loss of function is sometimes included in this list.

The mainstay of management for acute inflammation and pain management in healthy individuals is rest, ice, compression and elevation (RICE).

It is essential to identify the cause of the acute inflammation and, if possible, remove it and inform the patient of the cause and give advice on controlling pain.

CHRONIC WOUNDS (ULCERS)

Ulcers occur where a predisposing condition impairs the ability of the tissue to maintain integrity or heal from damage.

They may be superficial or deep, extending to bone, and may track under the tissues to have an extensive area of damage not visible on the skin's surface.

As with any break in the skin barrier, chronic wounds can become infected.

Assessment of chronic wounds

This should include the features of the skin generally, and that of surrounding the wound, the nature of the wound margins and base. The type of exudate in the wound and on the dressing must also be assessed and recorded for monitoring and evaluation purposes.

Swabs for culture and sensitivity may be taken if infection is present.

The wound may be measured across the diameter, or the margin traced on a sterile film; photographs can be stored in notes.

In general terms the tightly controlled sequential process of normal inflammation is disrupted and out of sequence in chronic wound healing.

Chronic wounds are frequently colonised by bacteria and healing can be delayed through infection when the bacteria present begin to have a pathological effect on tissue.

Management of chronic wounds

The primary aim of management is to prevent chronic wounds developing as they are painful and distressing for the patient and are costly to manage.

It is essential to recall that the patient's general health and drug therapy may inhibit an inflammatory response to infection, so the practitioner must be alert for other evidence of infection, such as increase in exudate, smell of exudate or increase in pain.

Management of chronic wounds is primarily according to the aetiology and site. Sites of increased mechanical stress must be protected and off-loaded with padding, orthoses, footwear adaptations or scotch cast boots and, if necessary, bed rest.

Chronic wounds change with time, so if copious exudate is present, then a highly absorptive dressing would be used, but when the wound changes to produce little exudate then a low-absorption dressing would be selected.

Patients may need to be seen daily or at intervals appropriate to the needs of management according to the nature of the wound, dressing used or whether they are re-dressing the lesion themselves.

Wounds healing by first intention will usually result in minimal scaring while those healing by second intention will develop noticeable scars.

Scarring on the dorsum of the foot causes little problem, unless it adheres to underlying tissue.

Plantar scarring can produce discomfort, as scar tissue does not have the biomechanical characteristics of normal skin.

Keloid is a much raised prominent scar which involves adjacent tissues and is seen in black skin ten times more frequently than in white skin.

Hypertrophic scarring is broader than normal scars and elevated above the surrounding skin; it is red, sometimes painful and sometimes with contracture.

BURNS

The skin can be damaged through thermal, photo and chemical burns.

Superficial burns involve only the epidermis, partial-thickness burns extend into the dermis. In full-thickness burns the epidermis and dermis are destroyed and muscle and bone may be involved.

Boiling water scalds and accidents with hot water bottles are frequent causes of burn injury to the foot.

Sunburn can cause severe immediate effects of pain and blistering as well as long-term skin malignancy.

The first aid for burns is to apply cold to the area, keeping it cool and covered to minimise risk of bacterial infection.

Chemical burns usually arise through spillage and inadvertent contact with the substance. This requires immediate irrigation of the site with water, hypertonic saline solution, buffer solution or neutralizer (if acidic use an alkali such as sodium bicarbonate, if alkali use a weak acid such as vinegar, if phenol use glycerine). If severe, hospital treatment will be required.

ATROPHY

Atrophic skin lacks nutrition owing to a poor blood supply through systemic or peripheral disorder, because of poor diet or malabsorption syndromes.

Atrophic skin is thin, mechanically weak and has poor viability (that is if it is damaged it will heal slowly, if at all).

Nails usually show changes due to atrophy.

CHILBLAINS AND CHILLING

This is a seasonal, vasospastic condition affecting the young and old; generally the mid-age group is less affected.

There may be an underlying medical condition complicating the problem.

Chilblains occur most commonly in the winter, are about 2 cm in diameter, are usually discoloured and may itch or be painful.

Initially the area of cold damage is white due to vasoconstriction. Later the site shows a bright red (erythematous) inflammatory reaction. A few hours later the site becomes swollen and bluish (cyanotic) with prolonged vasodilation.

Management requires minimising exposure to extremes of temperature and rapid temperature change, minimising mechanical stress and ensuring that an optimal healing rate is achieved.

Topical preparations can be applied according to the 'stage' of the chilblain; a cooling, soothing preparation can be used to control the inflammatory response in the erythematous stage, e.g. witch hazel. In the cyanotic phase, a rubefacient may help to stimulate superficial blood flow.

When the chilblain is broken it is essential to keep it free from infection and to protect tissues from mechanical stress by using padding and suitable dressings.

INFECTIONS AND THE SKIN

In health, the skin has very effective mechanisms for keeping infection out of the body, both through the primary skin barrier in the base of the stratum corneum and the immune system.

Bacterial and viral infections of the skin can develop if there is a break in the skin (wound) or if the pathogen is able to penetrate the skin barrier.

Wounds are frequently colonised by bacteria. Ulcers are chronic wounds which fail to heal in the expected time.

Fungal infections (e.g. tinea pedis) may have a secondary overlay of bacterial infection, and vice versa.

Bacterial infections

Systemic bacterial infection (septicaemia) can cause marked generalised erythema (redness), pruritus (itching) and scaling (scalded skin syndrome) in the skin.

Deep, localised and spreading infection (cellulitis) will show similar skin changes and pain perhaps also with lymphangitis (red lines of inflamed lymphatics) and lymphadenitis (lymph nodes inflamed).

Common skin bacteria and resultant conditions are *Staphylococcus aureus* and beta-haemolytic streptococci.

Features of cutaneous infections

Cutaneous bacterial infections have differing features according to the infecting pathogen and health of the host.

People who are immunocompromised, immunosuppressed or who have poor peripheral vascular supply and/or microcirculation will have a subdued response to infection and will show lessened or few signs of inflammation.

People with disorders such as diabetes mellitus are particularly susceptible to infection owing to the multisystem effects of these conditions.

The degree of inflammatory response, features of the lesion, and the nature of any exudate provide clinical diagnostic indicators of the pathogen.

Viral infections

Systemic viral infections can cause skin changes, e.g. HIV and Kaposi's sarcoma, Coxsackie virus (chickenpox) and papular, urticarial (itchy) rash.

Generally, skin viral infections are difficult to treat and a number of different strategies may be employed, including medicinal plant extracts.

Verrucae/warts

There are a number of human papilloma viruses (HPVs) which cause different clinical features and infect different body sites.

HPVs causing warts in the foot include:

HPV 1 – single, deep plantar warts
HPV2 – mosaic warts
HPV2, 4, 60 – raised warts.

Clinical features of verrucae (warts)

Single plantar wart (verruca)

The patient's age, lesion site and history will give clues to the viral aetiology. Very new single plantar warts may be mistaken for seed corns or a foreign body in the skin. Established verrucae have a rough, cauliflower-like surface, sometimes with black dots of thrombosed capillaries.

Mosaic warts look as though single, more shallow plantar warts have coalesced forming a mass of warty tissue. The site can vary – plantar, interdigital, peri- and subungual.

Management

Almost all wart treatments rely on destruction of the wart tissue with an increased opportunity for the HPV antigen to be presented to the immune system.

After any wart treatment patients must be given advice to remove the dressing if necessary (for example pain, suspected infection), have a warm, hypertonic saline footbath for about 5 minutes, re-dress with dry dressing and contact for an urgent appointment.

It is medicolegally and ethically essential to ensure that the patient is fully aware of this advice.

Topical preparations for wart treatment include monochloroacetic acid and trichloroacetic acid, which, for therapeutic classification purposes, are termed caustics.

Salicylic acid in strengths from 40 to 75% ointment in white soft paraffin (keratolytic) may be used alone or with monochloroacetic acid in saturated solution.

Trichloracetic acid may be used alone or usually with silver nitrate (75 or 95%), another caustic which forms a grey/brown/black eschar (scab-like cover).

For home use, there is a wide range of topical proprietary preparations that should be used as per the instructions supplied with the product.

Homeopathic methods include Thuja paint and herbals such as Kalanchoe leaves and tea tree oil.

Dermabrasion may also be used.

Electrosurgery

Often this method of treating warts is considered when all else fails as it entails giving a local anaesthetic, perhaps as an ankle block, followed by tissue excision and/or electrodesiccation and wound healing.

PARASITIC INFESTATIONS

As people travel more widely and insects travel with imported goods, so the range of parasites seen has altered.

Lice (Pediculosis) can infest different body sites and cause itching where they feed, as can scabies (Sarcoptes scabei) where they burrow in the skin.

Lumps and bumps and scratches in the skin which have no obvious explanation need to be looked at carefully along with a full history to help in diagnosis of parasites caught in tropical climates, e.g. tumbu bug and hookworm.

VITILIGO

The abnormal pigmentation in this condition is particularly obvious in dark-skinned people, and, as a differential diagnosis is leprosy, there may be some concern over the condition.

DISORDERS OF SWEATING

Hyperhidrosis or anhidrosis will cause changes in the skin's mechanical strength.

This will give rise respectively to moist fissures, usually interdigitally, and dry fissures around the heel.

Both forms of fissure may develop complications of superimposed fungal or bacterial infection, especially if the dermis is exposed.

Excess sweating may indicate a medical disorder, e.g. hyperthyroidism, while anhidrosis may suggest poor tissue nutrition, perhaps due to poor diet, malabsorption syndromes or peripheral vascular disease.

Management of hyperhidrosis includes use of sweat-absorbing insoles, changing and airing footwear frequently, and application of astringents and deodorants.

Management of anhidrosis involves restoring the normal stratum corneum water content by the use of emollients and barrier creams, and the application of hydrocolloid wafers or films.

FISSURES

Fissures can be moist or dry cracks in the epidermis at sites where the skin is under tension and may extend to and involve the dermis with potential for infection.

The common site for moist fissures is interdigitally and for dry fissures around the heel margins.

Management requires removal of the cause if possible (for example removal of the allergen, treating tinea pedis with an antifungal).

CORNS AND CALLUS

Callus (callosity, mechanically induced hyperkeratosis) is a yellowish plaque of hard skin and a corn is an inverted cone of similarly hard skin which is pushed into the skin.

Both conditions are associated with excess intermittent mechanical stress (shear, friction, pressure, torsion, and tension) which results in abnormal keratinisation.

Management of corns and callus

Successful management requires removal of the cause followed by treatment that is aimed at reducing pain and restoring normal skin function.

Poor-quality skin may be associated with medical disorder or poor nutrient intake. If the latter is a factor then referral for dietary advice may be relevant.

Podiatric symptomatic management involves callus reduction and corn enucleation with a scalpel to reduce pain.

Pads, adhesive or replaceable, can be used to reduce the duration of tissue loading and re-distribute mechanical stress, and manage pain (for example, holed or corn between the fourth and fifth toes).

BURSITIS

Inflammation of a congenital or adventitious (acquired) bursa is termed bursitis. This may be aseptic and acute, infected and acute, or chronic bursitis.

The clinical features (signs and symptoms) of inflammation of differing degrees of severity and history (including that of recent changes in footwear) should lead to the diagnosis.

Management requires removal of the cause of the problem, so if footwear is the cause then this must be changed to a type that fits the foot and does not rub. Foot function should be assessed for biomechanical abnormality and subsequent management (including orthoses and mobilisation to minimise shear and friction at this site, but without overloading adjacent tissues or body segments).

Anti-inflammatory preparations (orthodox treatments such as topical ibuprofen or complementary such as arnica, calendula) or physical therapies including low-level laser therapy, therapeutic ultrasound, or footbaths, can help in acute bursitis.

Chronic bursitis may benefit from a 're-sequencing' of the inflammatory process by use of topical rubefacients (for example weak iodine solution), therapeutic ultrasound (N.B. proximity of target tissue to bone) or contrast footbaths.

In all forms of bursitis, protection from mechanical stress is essential and may be achieved by changing or adapting footwear, providing replaceable or adhesive protective pads or covering with a polymer gel material that will absorb shear instead of the tissues.

The prognosis is good if diagnosis and management are correct.

THE SKIN AS AN INDICATOR OF PSYCHOLOGICAL DISTURBANCE

Picking nails to destruction (onychotillomania) may be considered problematic.

Cigarette burns on reachable areas of skin should also be observed carefully. This may be a sign of Munchausen's syndrome which can have many different forms.

Skin disorders may cause psychological problems, sometimes severe, as the failure of skin in cosmesis and function becomes intimately related to a sense of failure as a human.

THE NAIL IN HEALTH AND DISEASE

The human nail is a hard plate of densely packed keratinised cells which protects the dorsal aspect of the digits and greatly enhances fine digital movements of the hands.

The nail is a flat, horny structure, roughly rectangular and transparent.

The nail bed is normally seen through the plate as a pink area due to a rich vascular network.

In profile, the nail plate emerges from the proximal nail fold at an angle to the surface of the dorsal digital skin.

The proximal nail fold is an extension of the skin of the surface of the digit and lies superficial to the matrix, which is deeper in the tissues.

BLOOD SUPPLY AND INNERVATION

In the foot, the nail is supplied by two branches of the dorsal metatarsal artery and two branches of the plantar metatarsal artery.

They form an anastomosis at the terminal phalanx, the plantar arteries supplying the pad of the toe and the nail bed.

Innervation of the proximodorsal area of the nail and bed is provided by two small branches from the dorsal nerves (superficial peroneal (fibular), deep peroneal (fibular) and sural), while the medial and lateral plantar nerves provide a medial and lateral branch to each toe to supply the plantar skin, and extend to supply the anterodistal area of the nail bed and superficial skin.

Growth of the nail is continuous throughout life, the rate being greatest in the first two decades when the nail plate is thin.

The rate of growth decreases with age, and ultimately in the elderly the nail plate loses colour and may thicken and develop longitudinal ridges.

Nail growth is continuous throughout life, with peak rates of elongation in the group 10–14 years old and a steady decline in growth rate after the second decade; therefore, periodic cutting is necessary and incorrect performance of this task leads to onychocryptosis (ingrowing toe nail), one of the most painful conditions affecting nails.

INVOLUTION (PINCER, OMEGA NAIL)

This term describes a nail which increases in transverse curvature along the longitudinal axis of the nail, reaching its maximum at the distal part.

Tile-shaped nails often occur in association with yellow nail syndrome, affecting both fingers and toenails.

Plicatured nails occur where the surface of the plate remains flat while one or both edges of the nail form vertical parallel sides hidden by the sulcus tissue.

Pincer (omega, trumpet) nail dystrophy shows transverse curvature, which ranges from a minimal asymptomatic incurving to involution so marked that the lateral edges of the nail practically meet, forming a cylinder or roll; hence the names for this deformity.

Lateral compression of the nail may result in strangulation of the soft nail bed tissues and the formation of subungual ulceration as the circulation to the nail bed and matrix is reduced.

Treatment

In minor degrees, involution produces little or no discomfort and the main consideration is to ensure that the nail is cut so that it conforms to the length and shape of the toe.

More severe cases may be treated conservatively with careful clearing of the sulcus and the fitting of a nail brace.

Other derivatives of the nail brace are now available in plastic and are adhered to the nail directly.

Severe and painful involution is likely to require a unilateral or bilateral partial nail avulsion with destruction of the matrix.

If an underlying subungual exostosis is detected, this needs to be surgically excised.

ONYCHOCRYPTOSIS (INGROWING TOENAIL)

Onychocryptosis is a condition in which a spike, shoulder or serrated edge of the nail has pierced the epidermis of the sulcus and penetrated the dermal tissues.

The skin becomes red, shiny and tense and the toe appears swollen. There is throbbing pain, acute tenderness to the slightest pressure and a degree of localised hyperhidrosis.

The continued penetration of the nail spike prevents normal healing by granulation of the wound in the sulcus, and a prolific increase of granulation tissue is common (hypergranulation).

The most common predisposing factors are faulty nail cutting, hyperhidrosis and pressure from ill-fitting footwear, although any disease state which causes an abnormal nail plate may also be a factor.

If a nail is cut too short or the corners are cut obliquely, or if it is subjected to tearing, normal pressure on the underlying tissue is removed and without that resistance the tissue begins to protrude.

Tearing of the nails has a similar effect to cutting obliquely across the corners of the nail plate.

Treatment

If the onychocryptosis is uncomplicated by infection, the penetrating splinter may be removed.

It should then be packed firmly with sterile cotton wool or gauze, making sure that it is inserted a little way under the nail plate to maintain its elevation.

Betadine, applied to the packing and the toe is covered with a non-adherent sterile dressing and tubular gauze.

When onychocryptosis is complicated by infection and suppuration is present, it is important to remove the splinter of nail, facilitating drainage and allowing healing to take place.

Location and removal of the penetrating nail may cause considerable pain and a local anaesthetic should be given.

The patient should be advised to rest the foot and, if necessary, to cut away the upper of the slipper or shoe to remove all pressure from the toe.

The patient should return the following day for the renewal of dressings, and this must be continued until the sepsis is cleared.

If hypergranulation tissue is present, it may be excised.

Following this treatment the prognosis is good, but the patient must be given clear guidance on the predisposing factors so that they can avoid recurrence.

SUBUNGUAL EXOSTOSIS

Subungual exostosis is a small outgrowth of bone under the nail plate near its free edge or immediately distal to it.

As the outgrowth increases, the nail becomes elevated and displaced from the nail bed and the tumour may emerge from the free edge or destroy the nail plate.

The epidermis becomes stretched and thinned and takes on a bright red colour which blanches on pressure.

Temporary relief may be given by means of protective padding and advice on footwear, but surgical excision is always the most satisfactory treatment.

SUBUNGUAL HELOMA (CORN)

As the term implies, a subungual heloma is the development of a nucleated keratinised lesion under the nail plate. It is caused by trauma, which may be slight but prolonged, from shoes which are too short or too shallow, or sometimes from high-heeled shoes which produce abnormal pressure on the nail plate.

Treatment

If the heloma is near the free edge, an area of the nail plate can be removed to enable it to be enucleated.

Where the heloma is located towards the proximal half of the nail, it is necessary to reduce the nail thickness overlying the lesion with a nail drill.

Treatment may require to be repeated, especially if the heloma forms proximally. Modification of footwear may accommodate the deformity, but there are cases where nail surgery is indicated.

SUBUNGUAL MELANOMA

A variant of acral melanoma, this condition can be confused with subungual haematoma but careful examination of the physical signs and a detailed history will reduce the likelihood of misdiagnosis.

Most patients with melanoma have a fair complexion with light hair and blue or hazel-coloured eyes. The hallux and the thumb are the most likely sites to develop tumours.

Subungual melanoma manifests as an insidious pigmented spot in the matrix, nail bed or plate, or a longitudinal band of variable width in the nail plate. The latter often has a straight edge clearly seen along the plate. Either pigmented area may show one or more of several characteristics:

- variation in colour of the pigmented spot or band from brown to black; colour may be homogenous or irregular. It is seldom painful.
- pigment may spread to surrounding periungual tissues (Hutchinson's sign) and, although it is an important indicator of subungual melanoma, it is not a totally accurate predictor of melanoma.
- there is eventual dystrophy and destruction of the nail plate.

Diagnosis

Until recently diagnosis has been made almost exclusively following biopsy of the matrix and/or nail bed tissues, which is often painful and disfiguring.

Subungual melanoma has a poor prognosis, with up to 50% of patients dying within 5 years of the diagnosis.

ONYCHAUXIS (HYPERTROPHIED NAIL)

This is an abnormal but uniform thickening of the nail, increasing from the nail base to the free edge often accompanied by slight brown colour changes in the nail plate and enlargement of the sulci due to the thickened lateral edges of the nail.

Onychauxis occurs following damage to the nail matrix, for which there may have been one or more of several causes: a single major trauma or repeated minor traumas.

Fungal infection of the nails and chronic skin diseases or poor peripheral circulation can also be factors, especially in the elderly.

Irrespective of the cause, the nail should be reduced in size to as near normal as possible at each visit, in order to relieve the pain caused by pressure on the nail bed tissues.

If the patient is young and the condition is confined to one toenail only, avulsion of the nail and destruction of the matrix provide the most satisfactory treatment.

ONYCHOGRYPHOSIS (RAM'S HORN, OSTLER'S TOE)

As well as hypertrophy, there is gross deformity of the nail which develops into a curved or 'ram's horn' shape.

The commonest cause is a single major trauma. It is sometimes the result of neglect and the consequent increasing impaction from footwear against the lengthening nail.

Palliative treatment consists of reduction of the hypertrophy. In a young person, avulsion with matrix destruction is the most satisfactory method of treatment.

ONYCHOPHOSIS

A condition in which callus and/or the formation of a heloma occurs in the nail sulcus. It is caused by lateral pressure from constricting footwear or from an adjacent toe, or unskilled nail cutting; harsh probing of the sulcus may also lead to excessive thickening of the stratum corneum.

The callus can be cleared with a small scalpel and checked for the presence of corns, which must be enucleated. If removal is not possible it may be necessary to pack the sulcus with a keratolytic, such as 10–15% salicylic acid in collodium.

PARONYCHIA

Paronychia and onychia frequently occur together and are characterised by inflammation of the tissues surrounding the nail plate, the latter by inflammation of the matrix and the nail bed.

Any trauma to the toe might facilitate the entry of bacteria or a foreign body into the tissues which can predispose to paronychia.

There is always the possibility that the infection will become widespread, and, therefore, it is advisable to suggest that the patient consult a physician.

Once bacteria or other foreign bodies have gained access into the tissues, the natural defensive reaction of the body is to induce a local inflammatory response, which becomes red, swollen and extremely painful.

Paronychia should always be regarded as potentially serious and it must be ascertained whether the condition is acute or chronic.

Acute paronychia is mainly the result of local trauma and treatment is directed primarily towards the prevention of infection if this is not already present, and towards the reduction of inflammation and congestion.

If infection is present, the first principle is to promote drainage of any pus by means of a hot antiseptic footbath, repeated at home at 4-hourly intervals, or by surgically removing the nail plate. Arrangements should be made for the patient to obtain appropriate systemic antibiotic therapy from the doctor, while podiatric dressings continue at frequent intervals.

ONYCHIA

Onychia can, and often does, result from paronychia and the pathology is similar.

Immediate relief of acute pain will be obtained by removal of as much as necessary, or even all, of the nail plate to provide drainage of the underlying pus. Once this is achieved, the further treatment is the same as for paronychia.

ONYCHOLYSIS

Onycholysis is separation of the nail from its bed at its distal end and/or its lateral margins. It is more common in fingernails than toenails and affects women more frequently than men. Its aetiology is idiopathic as a result of systemic disease, cutaneous diseases, drug side effects, or local causes, such as trauma where only one nail will be affected.

Pathology

Separation of the nail is usually symptomless, but as the condition progresses the space becomes filled with hard keratinous material from the exposed nail bed.

If a systemic cause is suspected, the patient should be advised to consult a physician and the application of a suitable antifungal preparation at the active edge of the disease should be carried out.

ONYCHOMADESIS (ONYCHOPTOSIS, APLASTIC ANONYCHIA)

This is the spontaneous separation of the nail, beginning at the matrix area and quickly reaching the free edge and resulting in the arrest of nail growth, characterised by a Beau's line arising from trauma, generalised diseases, local inflammation, defective peripheral circulation or prolonged exposure to cold, or it may be an inherited disorder (dominant).

A newly formed subungual haematoma should be drained. For cases where trauma can be excluded, protect the nail with simple tubular gauze dressings.

ONYCHATROPHIA (ANONYCHIA)

Onychatrophia occurs when a nail of mature size undergoes partial or total regression.

Anonychia describes a nail which has failed to develop.

ONYCHORRHEXIS (REED NAIL)

This occurs as a series of narrow, longitudinal, parallel superficial ridges. The nail is very brittle and splitting at the free edge is common.

BEAU'S LINES

These are transverse ridges or grooves, which reflect a temporary retardation of the normal growth of the nail and move towards the free edge as the nail grows.

They are caused by any condition or disease which may temporarily affect nail production from the matrix.

No specific treatment, other than reassurance, is necessary.

HIPPOCRATIC NAILS (CLUBBING)

This is exaggerated longitudinal curvature of the nail, sometimes extending over the apex of the toe, and is associated with some long-standing pulmonary or cardiac disorder.

KOILONYCHIA (SPOON-SHAPED NAIL)

This occurs in infancy and more frequently in fingernails when the normal convex curvature is lost and, instead, it becomes slightly concave or spoon-shaped.

It is a temporary physiological condition, but there is a proven correlation between koilonychia and iron-deficiency anaemia.

ONYCHOMYCOSIS (TINEA UNGUIUM)

This is a fungal infection of the nail bed and nail plate.

Four types of fungal invasion

- Distal lateral subungual onychomycosis (DLSO) is the most common and often affects the skin of the palms and soles as well as the nails. Toenails are more frequently affected.
- Proximal subungual onychomycosis (PSO) is caused by moulds, e.g. *Scopulariopsis brevicaulis*.
- Superficial onychomycosis is most commonly due to *Trichophyton mentagrophytes var. interdigitale* and affects only toenails.
- Endonix onychomycosis is rare and is due to *Trichophyton soudanese* and *T. violaceum*. The nail plate is diffusely opaque and white and it is common for plantar tissues to be involved.

Fungally infected toenails often become thickened and quite brittle and in some cases take on a yellowish-brown colour. Left untreated, the nail becomes more friable and develops a 'worm-eaten' or porous appearance.

Of the dermatophytes associated with onychomycosis, the most frequently identified in practice are *Trichophyton rubrum* and *T. interdigitale*. Infection usually commences at the distal edge of the nail and gradually spreads over the entire nail plate and nail bed.

Management

Advice must emphasise the possible spread of the infection via towels, hosiery and shoes. Superficial onychomycosis can be treated with any topical antifungal agent; Amorolfine nail lacquer (5%) has proved successful if treatment is continuous for more than 6 months.

Dermatophyte onychomycosis requires systemic antifungal therapy.

LEUCONYCHIA

This involves white markings on the nail in lines (striata), dots (punctata) or extending over the entire nail plate and usually indicates minor trauma.

YELLOW NAIL SYNDROME

The rate of nail growth reduces greatly and sometimes almost ceases. All the nails become a yellowish-green colour.

The condition is almost always associated with some underlying respiratory or lymphoedema abnormality.

PTERYGIUM

Pterygium is the adhesion of the eponychium to the nail bed following destruction of the matrix due to diminished circulation or some systemic disease. The entire nail plate is eventually shed.

Chapter | **3** |

Dermatological conditions of the foot and leg

INFLAMMATORY SKIN DISEASES

Several chronic inflammatory skin diseases commonly involve the feet. A podiatrist should be able to recognise the clinical features of the most common skin diseases and be aware of appropriate management and referral criteria.

PSORIASIS AND RELATED DISORDERS

Psoriasis is a chronic inflammatory skin condition with a prevalence of about 2% of the UK population.

Any age group, including children, may be affected. There is clear evidence to suggest that susceptibility to psoriasis is inherited.

Types

- Chronic plaque psoriasis presents with circumscribed itchy patches of thick, scaly, red skin often prominent on the elbows, knees and scalp, although any body site can be affected
- Guttate psoriasis: multiple small patches of psoriasis erupt acutely after a streptococcal throat infection
- Erythrodermic psoriasis: a rare medical emergency in which more than 80% of the skin becomes red and inflamed
- Pustular psoriasis: numerous sterile pustules stud the surface of affected areas.

Aetiology

- Trauma (psoriasis appearing at sites of injury such as operative scars is called the Köbner phenomenon)
- Drugs, such as lithium or hydroxychloroquine
- Infection, particularly streptococcal pharyngitis which triggers guttate psoriasis
- Stress appears to be important in disease exacerbations in some patients.

Signs of psoriasis in the feet

- Pink or red plaques with a superficial layer of fine silvery white scales on the dorsal surface
- Hyperkeratotic, fissured skin on the plantar surface
- Nail dystrophy, including separation of the nail plate from the nail bed (onycholysis)
- Subungual hyperkeratosis
- Pitting of the nail plate which is more prominent on fingernails
- Psoriatic arthritis with pain and decreased mobility in the axial skeleton and the small joints of the hands and feet
- A rare mutilating form of arthritis can result in significant resorption of bone in the digits.

Differential diagnosis

- Eczema
- Lichen planus
- Pityriasis rubra pilaris
- Fungal infection.

Therapeutic management

- The severity of psoriasis can be assessed by the PASI (psoriasis area and severity index) score
- Regular emollients reduce scaling and fissuring
- Keratolytics such as 5% salicylic acid in Vaseline or 50% propylene glycol in water treat hyperkeratotic areas
- The numerous active topical treatments available include vitamin D analogues such as calcipotriol, topical steroids, coal tar-based preparations, dithranol (anthralin), an anthraquinone compound, and vitamin A-derived drugs (retinoids)
- Ultraviolet B (UVB) phototherapy or photochemotherapy using an oral or topical photoactive drug (a psoralen) in combination with ultraviolet A (PUVA)
- More severe cases may require treatment with drugs such as the oral retinoid acitretin, or immunosuppressive agents such as methotrexate or ciclosporin. The latter two agents in particular carry significant toxicity risks for bone marrow, liver or kidney, and all long-term systemic agents for psoriasis necessitate monitoring
- Patients with severe psoriasis not suitable for these drugs or who respond poorly may be treated with biological agents including TNF-alpha antagonists etantercept, infliximab and adalimumab. These agents carry the risks of immunosuppression, and are currently very expensive.

Palmoplantar pustular psoriasis (PPP)

- Chronic inflammatory disorder of the palms and soles
- Presents with red scaly hyperkeratotic palmar and plantar skin studded with sterile pustules
- Fresh pustules initially appear yellow and dry to leave brown discoloration
- Common in middle-aged women
- Strongly associated with cigarette smoking.

Differential diagnosis includes:

- acute infected eczema
- dermatophyte fungal infection
- Reiter's disease.

Treatment of PPP is similar to that of psoriasis but the disease is often resistant to many of the available therapeutic options.

Reiter's disease

- Reactive disorder in which arthritis, urethritis, conjunctivitis and inflammatory mucocutaneous disease are triggered by urogenital or gut infections
- Most commonly seen in young men and often follows *Chlamydia trachomatis* urethritis
- Classic cutaneous finding is keratoderma blenorrhagicum, a psoriasis-like eruption that affects the soles of the feet and may not appear for several months after the onset of arthritis and conjunctivitis
- Affected patients have thick, 'limpet-like' hyperkeratoses with a dull yellow discoloration or a more acute pustular rash
- Patients with active systemic disease may require treatment with immunosuppressive drugs
- Application of emollients and keratolytics may reduce the plantar keratoderma.

Pityriasis rubra pilaris (PRP)

A rare group of disorders of unknown aetiology characterised by:

- hyperkeratosis of hair follicles – spreads out to become confluent with patches of normal skin
- widespread erythema with a distinctive orange/yellow hue particularly prominent in the hyperkeratotic skin of the palms and soles
- palmoplantar keratoderma.

Treatment is with bland emollients, although many subsequently require the addition of systemic agents such as acitretin or methotrexate. Response to treatment is often poor, but the disease generally resolves spontaneously.

Eczema (dermatitis) and related disorders

An inflammatory skin disease caused by a number of factors. The terms eczema and dermatitis are synonymous.

Acute dermatitis is characterised by:

- redness
- scaling
- weeping often with vesiculation (tiny fluid-filled blisters).

Chronic dermatitis is characterised by:

- excoriation (scratch marks)
- thickening of the skin known as lichenification.

Common categories of eczema include:

- atopic eczema. A common, chronically relapsing skin disease with a genetic predisposition associated with the other atopic diseases, asthma and hay fever. Onset in infancy and about 60% of children are clear of dermatitis by the age of 10 years. Treatment is with emollients and topical corticosteroids

- contact dermatitis. Caused by a hypersensitivity reaction to specific allergens (*allergic contact dermatitis*), sensitised (allergic) to a wide variety of allergens present in footwear, hosiery or topical medicaments, or as a non-specific reaction to irritants (*irritant contact dermatitis*), such as soaps, detergents and even water. Diagnosis of allergens is by patch testing
- stasis and varicose eczema. Chronic venous or lymphatic insufficiency may cause dermatitis
- pompholyx. Acute vesicular type of dermatitis that affects the palms (cheiropompholyx) and soles (podopompholyx)
- juvenile plantar dermatosis. Irritant plantar dermatitis that occurs almost exclusively in children. The differential diagnosis includes allergic contact dermatitis and fungal infection. Treatment is with emollients, leather footwear and cork insoles.

Lichen planus

This is an intensely itchy inflammatory skin condition, immunologically mediated. It may be associated with adverse reactions to drugs.

Signs and symptoms

- Itchy, polygonal, violaceous, flat-topped papules covered with superficial white lines known as Wickham's striae
- Papules may coalesce into plaques
- Lesions can appear in lines of trauma (Köebner phenomenon)
- Rash can affect any body site; wrists and ankles are particularly common
- Nail dystrophy
- Scarring alopecia
- Plantar lesions are often not characteristic of lichen planus lesions at other sites
- Disease may range from a few discrete papules at the margin of the foot to widespread hyperkeratosis with fissuring and ulceration
- Usually a self-limiting disease.

The treatment for widespread, severe disease is systemic steroids, although more limited disease may respond well to potent topical steroids. Hyperkeratotic plantar involvement should be treated with combinations of keratolytics.

Ichthyosis

'Dry skin' or ichthyosis of varying degrees is common in the population. Skin is rough and scaly.

Inherited palmoplantar keratodermas

Plantar skin is characterised by a markedly thickened outer horny layer, or stratum corneum.

The keratodermas can be divided into inherited or acquired keratodermas. Inherited keratodermas are genetic skin diseases characterised by variable degrees of palmar and plantar hyperkeratosis.

Aetiology

- Mutations in a variety of mainly structural genes of the epidermis.

Clinical features (Table 3.1)

Table 3.1 Examples of inherited palmoplantar keratoderma and their causes (Judge et al. 2004)

PATTERN OF KERATODERMA	DISEASE	INHERITANCE	OTHER FEATURES	GENETIC BASIS
Diffuse				
	Epidemolytic PPK (Vörner)	Autosomal dominant: well-demarcated symmetrical involvement of palms and soles; marked redness at edge of keratoderma; epidermolysis present on histology	No	Mutation in keratin 9 gene
	Mutilating keratoderma with ichthyosis	Autosomal dominant: onset in infancy; honeycomb-like keratoderma; constrictions may form on digits	Ichthyosis	Mutation in loricrin gene
	Mutilating keratoderma with deafness (Vohwinkel)	Autosomal dominant: onset in infancy; honeycomb-like keratoderma; constrictions may form on digits	Hearing loss	Specific mutation in gap Junction B 2 (connexin 26) gene
Focal and striate				
	Focal non-epidermolytic Palmoplantar keratoderma	Autosomal dominant: onset in infancy	Oral leukokeratoses	Keratin 16

Continued

Table 3.1 Examples of inherited palmoplantar keratoderma and their causes (Judge et al. 2004)—cont'd

PATTERN OF KERATODERMA	DISEASE	INHERITANCE	OTHER FEATURES	GENETIC BASIS
	Pachyonychia congenita Type I (Jadassohn–Lewandowsky) Type II (Jackson–Lawler)	Autosomal dominant: hyperkeratosis over pressure points; palms and soles. No associated malignancy	Type I; orogenital, laryngeal and follicular hyperkeratosis; nail and hair abnormalities. Type II; nail and teeth abnormalities; cysts and bushy eyebrows	Type I; keratin 6 or 16 gene mutation. Type II; keratin 6b or 17 gene mutation
	Howell–Evans syndrome (tylosis)	Focal PPK; perifollicular papules	Oral hyperkeratosis; oral and oesophageal carcinoma	Linked to 17q24
	Striate keratoderma (Siemens)	Autosomal dominant: onset in infancy; extension onto elbows and knees	No	Mutation in desmoglein 1 or Desmoplakin
Punctate	Punctate PPK, (Buschke–Fischer–Brauer)	Autosomal dominant: develops at ages 12–30 yrs; multiple tiny punctate keratoses on palms and soles coalescing to diffuse keratoderma over pressure points	Variable nail abnormalities	Unknown

Judge MR, McLean WHI, Munro CS 2004 Disorders of keratinisation. In: Rook's Textbook of Dermatology, 7th Edn., Burns, Breathnach, Cox, Griffiths (eds). Blackwell, Oxford, Pp 34.1–34.111

Treatment

- Use of topical keratolytics such as salicylic acid 5–10% in white soft paraffin
- 35–70% propylene glycol
- Occlusion with polythene increases the efficacy of keratolytics
- Scalpel debridement or abrasion with a pumice stone
- Oral vitamin A derived drugs (retinoids), but may result in increased pain in affected skin
- Surgery has an occasional role for patients with focal keratoderma
- Keratoderma may be complicated by dermatophyte fungal infections.

Acquired keratodermas

- Keratoderma climactericum:
  - affects obese post-menopausal women
  - presents with erythema and hyperkeratosis over the heel and forefoot
  - is often asymptomatic, although pain on walking can be a problem if there is extensive involvement
  - has been described in younger women following oophorectomy
  - is treated with emollients and keratolytics.

Acrokeratosis paraneoplastica (Bazex's syndrome)

A rare cause of acquired keratoderma associated with some internal malignancies with keratoderma on hands and feet. Successful treatment of the underlying malignancy often leads to resolution of the disorder.

Keratoderma and hypothyroidism

Palmar and plantar hyperkeratoses have been reported in association with hypothyroidism. Treatment with thyroxine replacement may result in clinical improvement.

BLISTERING DISORDERS

Aetiology

- Bacterial or viral infections
- Insect bites
- Inflammatory skin disorders
- Traumatic blistering of the feet
- Poorly fitting or inappropriate footwear
- Rare skin disorders that are characterised by blistering as a result of inherited abnormalities.

Epidermolysis bullosa: the inherited mechanobullous disorders

Epidermolysis bullosa (EB) encompasses a spectrum of disorders characterised by skin fragility and blistering following mild mechanical trauma. Recent research into EB has identified the molecular basis for a number of the diseases, opening up the possibility for pre-natal diagnosis and gene-targeted therapy in the future.

EB can be broadly divided into three groups of diseases:

- in *EB simplex* the plane of cleavage is through the basal keratinocyte layer of the epidermis. Variants include the *Weber–Cockayne* variety in which non-scarring blisters predominantly affect palmar and plantar skin. The condition typically worsens in warm weather, particularly in childhood.
- in *junctional EB* separation is at the upper level of the dermo-epidermal junction. Skin and oral mucosa may be affected by blisters that heal with scars.
- in *dystrophic EB* separation is below the lower level of the dermo-epidermal junction. Blistering starts in infancy and affected patients have a relentlessly progressive course with scarring following minimal trauma. Growth retardation and anaemia may result from blistering and strictures in the oesophagus.

Autoimmune blistering disorders

Disease mediated by auto antibodies against target antigens in the epidermis or its basement layer results in increased skin fragility or blistering:

- *bullous pemphigoid* is the commonest autoimmune blistering disorder
- the whole epidermis lifts off producing an intact firm blister
- on the feet the blisters may be more vesicular resembling those of pompholyx
- in the various forms of pemphigus, antibodies are directed against adhesion molecules within the epidermis and the result is friable blisters or erosions
- common in the elderly
- treatment is aggressive with high doses of oral corticosteroids or other immunosuppressive agents.

TUMOURS

Tumour in Latin simply means a swelling. These are divided into benign or malignant. Some normally benign lesions may become malignant. Some apparently aggressive malignancies may spontaneously involute. A basal cell carcinoma in the skin may be locally malignant and destructive, but virtually never metastasises.

Classification of skin tumours (Table 3.2)

Table 3.2 Examples of inherited palmoplantar keratoderma and their causes

TUMOUR TYPE	DEGREE OF MALIGNANCY	EXAMPLES
Epidermal tumours	Benign	Seborrhoeic keratoses
	Premalignant	Bowen's disease
	Malignant	Basal cell carcinoma
		Squamous cell carcinoma

Table 3.2 Examples of inherited palmoplantar keratoderma and their causes—cont'd

TUMOUR TYPE	DEGREE OF MALIGNANCY	EXAMPLES
Cutaneous metastatic tumours	Benign	Freckle
		Lentigo
Pigmented skin tumours		Congenital naevus
		Benign acquired naevus
		Speckled and lentiginous naevus
		Becker's naevus
		Spitz naevus
	Premalignant	Dysplastic naevus
	Malignant	Malignant melanoma
Epidermal and dermal naevi	Benign	Pyogenic granuloma
		Glomus tumour
Vascular tumours	Malignant	Kaposi's sarcoma
Fibrous tumours	Benign	Acquired fibrokeratoma
		Dermatofibroma
	Malignant	Dermatofibrosarcoma protuberans
Adnexal tumours	Benign	Eccrine poroma
Other structures	Benign	Leiomyoma (smooth muscle)
		Subungual exostosis (bone)
		Myxoid cyst (joint)
		Ganglion (joint)
		Bursitis (joint)
		Piezogenic pedal papules (fat)
		Neurofibromatosis (nerve)

Aetiology

- The cause of many skin tumours is unknown
- Areas of long-continued skin damage may undergo malignant transformation:
  - leg ulcers
  - burns
  - tuberculosis infections
  - X-radiation
  - excess exposure to ultraviolet radiation, mainly of the 280–320 nm range
- Papilloma virus (especially types 16/18)
- Herpes virus is established in some cases of Kaposi's sarcoma
- Retrovirus in some T-cell lymphomas
- UV-induced.

Epidermal tumours

Seborrhoeic keratosis

Synonyms: senile or seborrhoeic wart, basal cell papilloma.

- Seborrhoeic keratoses are some of the commonest tumours.
- Incidence increases with advancing age.

- They tend to cluster on the trunk but any body surface, including the feet, can be involved.
- Stucco keratosis generally affects the legs and ankles.

Aetiology

This is unknown.

Clinical features

- Commonest type of seborrhoeic keratosis is found on the trunk
- Initially small papular lesions with a slight increase in pigmentation
- Become larger, usually up to about 1 cm in diameter, tend to darken, sometimes until they are almost black
- Can become very large: ≥10 cm
- Edge is distinct and may slightly overhang the surrounding normal skin
- Degree of pigmentation is variable but is usually homogeneous throughout any individual lesion
- Surface is rough and wart-like and at times can become extremely heaped up and thickened
- Small circumscribed round areas on the surface are characteristic and known as horn cysts
- Surface colour is matt and lacklustre
- On palpation they can feel rather greasy
- Horn cysts give it a warty feel
- On the extremities lesions tend to be flatter
- Some can be irritated by clothing, etc., and secondary infection can supervene
- May spontaneously resolve
- Normally several other lesions are present
- Massive numbers can erupt rapidly. This is called the sign of Leser–Trélat
- Stucco keratosis is the name given to a type usually seen on the legs and ankles. Usually white or grey in appearance and smaller, rarely exceeding 3–4 mm.

Diagnosis

- By careful examination
- Lesion may be confused with viral warts and other hyperkeratotic lesions
- Various pigmented lesions may need to be excluded
- Histological diagnosis – keratinocytes resembling basal cells gather in the epidermis
- Increased numbers of melanocytes may contribute to the darkening colour
- Concentric whorls of keratin form the keratin cysts.

Treatment

- Usually indicated for cosmetic reasons
- Lesion is catching and becoming irritated
- A short application of liquid nitrogen
- Curette off easily
- Able to obtain histology if there is diagnostic doubt.

Bowen's disease

Bowen's disease is an intradermal carcinoma in situ which can slowly progress towards a squamous cell carcinoma.

Aetiology

- Sun damage
- Arsenic exposure
- Papilloma virus.

Clinical features

- Bowen's has a preponderance to affect the lower leg
- Predilection for the head and neck
- Slowly enlarging reddish, scaly patch with definite margins. Can be mistaken for psoriasis
- Some of the patches may be more crusted or raised.

Differential diagnosis

- Basal cell carcinoma
- Squamous cell carcinoma
- Malignant melanoma
- Eczema
- Psoriasis
- Rarely, a nail bed or periungual variant.

Histology

- Entire epidermis is replaced by very abnormal-looking keratocytic cells
- Exhibits nuclear atypia with numerous abnormal mitoses
- Premature keratinisation which leads to intraepidermal pink horn cysts
- Basement membrane remains intact until malignancy supervenes.

Treatment

- In the early stages it can respond to the topical application of 5-fluorouracil ('Efudix')
- Cryotherapy
- Photodynamic therapy
- Topical imiquimod
- Excision.

Basal cell carcinoma

Basal cell carcinoma (synonyms: rodent ulcer, basal cell epithelioma) is the commonest skin tumour, certainly of the white races. They are extremely rare on the foot, especially the plantar surface. A certain number occur on the leg.

Clinical features

- The incidence of basal cell carcinoma increases with age
- The commonest site is on the face, which may suggest a solar aetiology
- Small lesion developing and extending very slowly over months or years
- Crusts from time to time
- The crust comes off with a little bleeding in repeated cycles

- Slow peripheral growth
- Round or oval outline with a raised or rolled border
- Border pinkish and slightly nodular, and is likened to a string of pearls
- Dilated telangiectatic vessels at edge
- Centre may ulcerate or be more raised and dome-shaped
- Locally they may be very large and destructive, eroding down to the deep structures.

Differential diagnosis

- Those on the lower leg can be less characteristic and diagnosis may be difficult:
  - bowen's disease
  - squamous cell carcinoma
  - malignant melanoma
  - vascular lesions
  - metastasise rarely
  - multiple lesions may occur and some may be the naevoid basal cell carcinoma syndrome (Gorlin's syndrome). With reference to the feet and hands, small pits or depressions may be seen on the plantar and palmar surfaces.

Histology

- Cells resembling those of the basal cell layer or appendages appear to 'bud' down from that layer.
- They form spherical masses of very uniform cells in the dermis.
- Characteristically the cells at the periphery of these spheres line up in a regular arrangement known as pallisading.
- The masses are surrounded by a fibrous stroma.

Treatment

- Most are best surgically excised
- Curettage
- Cryotherapy
- Photodynamic therapy
- Radiation
- Topical imiquimod.

Squamous cell carcinoma

Cutaneous squamous cell carcinoma arises from skin keratinocytes. It is the second commonest skin tumour after basal cell carcinoma. It may affect any area of the skin. It is relatively rare on the foot. A rare variant, verrucose carcinoma, targets the foot.

Aetiology

- Age
- Inability to naturally protect the skin, such as albinos with no pigment
- Impairment of DNA repair mechanisms as in xeroderma pigmentosum
- HIV/AIDS
- Some skin lesions are known to be pre-malignant, for example Bowen's disease (carcinoma in situ) or actinic keratoses
- Areas of chronic irritation, including leg ulcers, may progress to squamous cell carcinoma

- Human papilloma
- Contamination with tars, heavy mineral oils, hydrocarbons, etc.
- Exposure to ultraviolet radiation
- X-radiation is also carcinogenic
- Repeated damage from radiant heat may provoke erythema ab igne and rarely may progress to squamous cell carcinoma
- Arsenic exposure.

Clinical features

Squamous cell carcinoma may present in very many different ways. Thus in any unusual or non-responsive skin condition the possibility of it should be borne in mind, otherwise it may be missed:

- chronic skin diseases such as actinic keratosis, Bowen's disease, leg ulcers, burns, etc., have potential to transform to malignancy
- presents in a sun-exposed area but no site is immune
- starts as a reddish plaque, mimicking eczema or dermatitis
- edges tend to be irregular and the lesion indurated
- commence or progress to a nodule of variable size, the surface of which is usually raw and does not epithelialise
- may ooze serosanguinous fluid
- some squamous cell carcinomas ulcerate:
  - ulcer is irregular in shape with undermined ragged edges
  - the base is covered with a dirty yellowish green slough
- squamous cell cancers of the nail are often misdiagnosed
- the feet are less commonly affected than the hand

The vast majority of squamous cell carcinomas are only locally aggressive, but if neglected can spread to the draining lymph nodes and to other areas. Head, neck, genital and large tumours all spread more quickly.

Squamous cell carcinoma variant; verrucose carcinoma of the foot

Synonyms: epithelioma or carcinoma cuniculatum:

- verrucose carcinoma may appear at any site
- has a predilection for the plantar aspect of the foot
- initially it may resemble a simple verruca plantaris
- progresses relatively slowly and may become nodular
- differential diagnosis would include many nodular foot lesions
- the tumour increases, becomes soggy and foul-smelling
- it has a marked tendency to burrow under the skin surface, sinuses appearing at a slightly distant site from the main lesion
- rarely metastasise.

Histology

- In squamous cell carcinoma the epidermal cells are malignant
- Large, well-differentiated cells with some individual cell keratinisation to bizarre, abnormal cells with little or no resemblance to epidermal cells
- While in situ, they are contained by the basement membrane to within the epidermis
- 'Break through' into the dermis, initially often in fine filaments, but later in broad masses
- Verrucose carcinoma is a well-differentiated tumour

- Clinical suspicion should override an apparently normal biopsy. The cancer may not have manifested itself histologically or the sample may have missed the diagnostic part.

Treatment

- Prevention should be practised control of ultraviolet exposure, radiation, etc.
- Potentially pre-malignant lesions should be treated
- Monitor those at risk for genetic reasons
- Monitor the immunosuppressed and transplanted patient
- Immunisation programmes to reduce the future incidence of genital skin and cervical cancers
- Established squamous cell carcinoma, surgical excision with histological confirmation
- If there is suspicion of lymph-node involvement a suitable dissection should be undertaken
- In the few patients where surgery is not an option:
  - cryotherapy
  - laser
  - photodynamic therapy
  - intralesional injections.

Cutaneous metastatic disease

Neoplasms beginning in another tissue may spread to the skin by direct extension or as local or distant metastases. These lesions may occur in a patient with known malignant disease or be the first manifestation of the underlying tumour. Skin malignancies themselves, notably melanoma, may also metastasise to other areas of the skin.

Clinical features

- The non-skin tumours that most commonly spread to the skin are:
  - breast
  - colon and rectum
  - ovary
  - prostate.
- There is a wide range of skin lesions:
  - small nodules are the commonest. They often appear to be under the skin, pushing up from below and splaying out the normal skin markings
  - indurated erythema
  - telangiectic plaques
  - non-healing ulcers
  - skin metastasis from another skin tumour will often mimic the original tumour. Malignant melanoma is the commonest cause.

Treatment

The treatment is essentially that of the primary lesion. In a few instances treatment of the skin lesion by surgery, radiation or chemotherapy may be considered.

Pigmented skin lesions

Skin colour is largely, though not entirely, due to melanin pigment produced by melanocytes.

Naevus

A naevus is a non-malignant growth. Pigmented naevi (moles) form a large group.

Classification of pigmented naevi

- Freckles
- Lentigo
- Congenital naevus
- Benign acquired naevus
- Becker's naevus
- Spitz naevus
- Malignant melanoma.

Freckles

These are common, especially in red-haired persons of Celtic extraction. They are up to 2–3 mm and tend to be familial. Freckles require ultraviolet radiation to develop and usually appear in sun-exposed areas at the age of 3–5 years. Treatment is unnecessary, though these populations are statistically more liable to malignant melanomas.

Lentigo

Lentigos are flat, brownish/black lesions, of which the most common are 'age' or 'liver' spots on the dorsa of the hands are examples. They may be induced by sun (solar or actinic changes). They may respond to cryotherapy.

The sun bed and PUVA lentigos indicate skin damage and such patients may be at later risk to develop malignant melanoma.

Congenital melanocytic naevus

By definition, congenital melanocytic naevi should be present at birth and about 1% of neonates have these. However, similar lesions can develop up to a few years post partum and may be included under this title.

Clinical features

- Congenital melanocytic naevi are usually brown to black in colour.
- The skin marking can be seen traversing the lesion.
- In many cases, hair of an inappropriate terminal type will develop.
- The surface of the lesion may be smooth, ranging to warty or lobular.
- An irregular edge may cause concern but the pigmentation is relatively homogeneous.
- They grow disproportionately slowly with age compared with the increase in body size.

Treatment

- The incidence of congenital melanocytic naevi developing malignancy is disputed but the larger they are the more likely is this complication
- Large congenital melanocytic naevi of the extremities seem to be immune from malignancy
- Serial photography is advocated
- Small lesions may be excised for cosmetic reasons

- The larger the lesion, the more disfiguring it is, but the more difficult it is to excise
- Regular monitoring and cosmetic camouflage.

Acquired melanocytic naevus

An acquired melanocytic naevus is an abnormality. They affect both sexes and appear at intervals throughout life. Small numbers present, peaking in incidence around the teens, then falling off in old age.

Clinical features

- Occur in both sexes
- Increased prevalence in black skin
- Junctional naevi are the commonest on palms, soles and genitalia
- They are usually flat
- A few millimetres in diameter
- Round or oval shape
- Colour varies from brown to dark black
- Compound naevi are usually dome-shaped papules with a light to dark colour
- Coarse hair may grow through the lesion
- Occasionally there can be a circle of increased pigmentation around the periphery
- The nail matrix may be affected by junctional or compound naevi. Longitudinal melanonychia may occur.

Intradermal naevi

With the disappearance of the junctional component, pigmentation tends to fade. In intradermal naevi, the lesion is often a flesh-coloured papule. Hair may grow through it.

Treatment

- It is manifestly impossible to remove all naevi
- Surgical removal can be carried out for cosmetic reasons
- Surgical removal if constant irritation occurs
- The patient must be aware that formal surgical excision will inevitably result in a scar
- Some protuberant lesions may be improved by a shave biopsy.

Speckled and lentiginous naevus

Speckled and lentiginous naevi are considered relatively rare.

Clinical features

The lesion usually develops in childhood on the extremities, but other areas can be affected. A light-brown macular area may measure up to 10 cm in diameter. Spots which may be very dark develop within this.

Treatment

- There are sporadic reports of malignant melanoma developing. If surgically reasonable, excision may be the best option

- Close monitoring with photographic records should be undertaken
- Laser treatment.

Becker's naevus

Becker's naevus is a fairly common lesion, occurring in about 1 in 2000 young men and one-fifth of that in females. It is pigmented but there are few or no changes in the melanocytes.

Clinical features

- It usually appears in the late teens or early adult life, gradually becoming more obvious.
- The usual site to be involved is the shoulder, but other areas, including the leg, have been described.
- It is often a large area (over 20 cm) with a markedly indented outline.
- Within it, there can be white island areas about the size of a fingerprint.
- Normally, coarse, darkish hairs develop within the patch.

Treatment

Becker's naevus is usually too large for surgical removal. Cosmetic camouflage appears to be the solution.

Spitz naevus

Spitz naevus is a benign melanocytic lesion similar to a compound naevus. The histology can be very similar to that of malignant melanoma and pathologists asked to look at it without an adequate history may diagnose the latter.

Clinical features

- Spitz naevi usually occur in young people up to the age of 20.
- Head, neck and leg are common locations.
- They are usually asymptomatic dome-shaped firm nodules, which are pink, red or tan in colour.

Treatment

Complete excision is best.

Dysplastic naevi

Synonym: clinically atypical naevus. Some patients have naevi, often multiple, which exhibit clinical and/or histological features which are unusual and worrying. They prove a difficult management problem.

Clinical features

- These are clinically atypical lesions and the great concern is to try to differentiate them from malignant melanoma.
- They may occur in any site, either singly or sometimes in vast numbers.
- They tend to be larger than benign naevi, often more than 5 mm in diameter.
- They are roughly round or oval, with some asymmetry.
- The border is irregular but often fuzzy rather than sharper, larger projections of the malignant melanoma.
- There may be a collarette of increased pigmentation.

- Colour variegation within the lesion is common but more 'twin tone' in contradistinction to the multiple variations seen in malignant melanoma.
- The areas of pigmentation have more regular edges.
- Skin markings are usually uninterrupted.
- There is an increased chance of melanoma developing most marked with multiple lesions and a family history of malignant melanoma.

Treatment

- Any dysplastic naevi which cause clinical concern should be excised, along the same lines as for malignant melanoma.
- If there is little concern no treatment is required.
- Multiple lesions and a family history of malignant melanoma require regular supervision.
- General photographic views plus individual close-ups are invaluable.

Malignant melanoma of the skin

A cutaneous malignant melanoma arises from melanocytes in the epidermis. Similar tumours may occur in other tissues, e.g. the eye. It is vitally important that early diagnosis is made when a cure can be effected. Diagnosis in the later stages greatly increases the chance of death. There has been a tremendous increase in the incidence of the tumour in the last 50 to 60 years.

Aetiology

- Sun exposure
- A single or a few burning episodes in the child or the young adult seems to be more provocative than longer-term outdoor unprotected activity
- The red-headed, freckled, fair-skinned are more at risk
- Higher incidence in outdoor workers
- In a few cases, there is an apparent hereditary tendency to develop malignant melanoma
- Patients with some pre-existing pigmented lesions are at more risk of malignant melanoma.

Clinical features

- Some malignant melanomas produce little or no pigment and are termed hypo- or amelanotic melanomas. They pose particular difficulties in diagnosis
- A careful history and meticulous examination in a good light are essential
- A changing lesion should be paid particular attention if the following are observed:
  - irregularity
  - increasing size
  - bleeding
  - discharging
  - itching.
- An ABCD checklist:
  - A = asymmetry of the outline
  - B = border irregularity
  - C = colour variegation
  - D = diameter enlargement
- Very early lesions will not have developed the above

- The prognosis depends vitally on the thickness of the melanoma
- A horizontal growth pattern is termed a superficial spreading melanoma and has a reasonably good outlook in general
- A vertical growth pattern rapidly spreads into the lymphatics and blood vessels, metastasising earlier with a poorer prognosis. These are termed nodular melanomas.

Clinical types of melanoma

- Lentigo malignant melanomas are slow-growing lesions, usually on the face, commonly in the elderly:
    - a flat lentiginous lesion
    - irregular border
    - colour variegation slowly extending
    - a central nodule may develop
    - aggressive and spreading
- Superficial spreading melanoma. This is the most commonly encountered type in the Caucasian:
    - occurs on any site
    - more likely on the male back or the female leg
    - irregular features
    - raised with palpable areas indicating a thicker, nodular type indicates a poorer prognosis
    - change in the central colour to a bluish colour
    - central clearing may occur, usually meaning the tumour is growing deeper and the alteration in colour is due to a physical light-scattering effect
- Nodular melanoma. Growth can be rapid and is likely to be hypo- or amelanotic:
    - a vascular lesion is a common misdiagnosis due to the raised, friable, oozing nature
    - there may be a ring of pigmentation on careful examination
- Acral lentiginous melanoma. This is relatively uncommon in whites but more common in blacks and orientals:
    - a flat lentiginous area on palms, soles or around nails
    - progresses in size more rapidly than other malignant melanomas
    - ultimately develops nodules
    - has a poorer prognosis than other melanomas. May be due to a longer delay in diagnosis on a relatively non-visualised foot in the average patient
- Subungual melanomas:
    - are a particularly difficult type to differentiate from benign melanonychia or subungual haematomas
    - the melanoma is usually proximal and if the pigmentation involves the posterior nail fold (Hutchinson's sign) this is more ominous
    - thickness of the malignant melanoma is important. The pathologist has a vital role to play in the measurable assessment of this. Originally, this was done by measuring the invasion of the tumour in relation to other anatomical structures of the dermis. These were known as Clark's levels I–V:
        - I – only in the epidermis (i.e. in situ)
        - II – just into upper dermis
        - III – significantly into upper dermis
        - IV – in deeper reticular dermis
        - V – into deep fat.

This can be difficult on certain areas, particularly acral sites and a micrometer measurement known as the Breslow thickness is more often used. Melanomas under 0.75 mm are considered to have a good prognosis, over that the outlook declines with increasing thickness.

Treatment

- Prevention by removing all known removable causes
- Advice on the dangers of sun exposure
- Persons at risk from genetic problems require careful monitoring
- In the suspected malignant melanoma fast-track referring is essential
- On positive diagnosis rapid and adequate excision is paramount
- The exact surgical clearance margins are; the thicker the lesion, the wider should be the margins
- Regional lymph nodes, if involved, are excised
- Chemotherapy.

Vascular tumours

Pyogenic granuloma

These are common lesions which usually follow an injury which may not be remembered by the patient.

Clinical features

- A friable vascular lesion develops rapidly at the site of a previous injury
- Multiple lesions may be triggered in severe acne
- Paronychia
- A thorn or pinprick injury followed by the development of a mushroom-type lesion
- Bleeds on the slightest touch
- Nail-fold lesions are constrained and lose their mushroom appearance
- Lesions vary in size, usually up to 1 cm
- Epithelialisation can be seen in long-established pyogenic granulomas
- Some spontaneously involute.

Diagnosis

- Pyogenic granuloma is usually an easy diagnosis to make and usually responds to treatment.

  Differential diagnosis:
- malignant melanoma, especially the a- or hypo-melanotic type
- bowen's disease
- squamous cell carcinoma
- verrucose carcinoma
- eccrine poroma
- metastatic lesions may confuse.

Histology

- Circumscribed lesion
- Contains multiple capillaries, some very dilated
- Considerable proliferation of endothelial cells
- At the base, the epidermis tends to grow, leading to a collarette constricting the lesion and contributing to the 'mushroom stalk'.

Treatment

- Curettage
- Histological examination
- Formal excision.

Glomus tumour

Glomus tumours are rare and originate from the cells of smooth muscle whose normal function is to regulate temperature by acting as valves on arteriovenous anastomotic shunts which are most profuse on the digits. Glomus tumours are commonest on the digits, although a multiple variety occurs.

Clinical features

- Preceding trauma
- Occurs at any age
- Affects either sex
- A small purplish nodule develops about 5 mm diameter
- Under the nail, can give it a purplish colour
- The usual cardinal symptom is pain triggered by minor pressure or temperature reduction
- Confirmed in early stages by the use of magnetic resonance imaging
- Multiple lesions are called glomangiomas and occur as scattered blue dermal nodules.

Treatment

Removal of a single lesion by surgery is the best option. Multiple ones may be considered for laser treatment.

Kaposi's sarcoma

Kaposi's sarcoma was originally described in 1872. It is now much more common and various types are recognised. These include:

- a sporadic (or classic) type
- African endemic
- immunosuppressive drug-induced
- HIV related.

Aetiology

Numerous cases in association with immunosuppression due to drugs or HIV led to further study and human herpes virus number 8 has been found in all forms of the disease.

Clinical features

- The classic or sporadic form mainly affects males of over 60 years.
- The most affected site is the leg or foot, although rarely lymph node and internal organs can be affected.
- The African type has various forms, ranging from one similar to the classic, through to a florid rapidly disseminating systemic variety. It can affect all ages.
- Kaposi's sarcoma is associated with immunosuppression.

- Kaposi's sarcoma associated with AIDS/HIV tends to be a very aggressive disease – survival time is up to 3 years. Systemic involvement affecting lymph nodes, GI tract and lungs.
- The original skin changes of multiple bluish tumours look rather like a bunch of grapes, located mainly on the extremities. Macular, papular, nodular and plaque forms have all been noted. Most forms have a purplish colour.

The differential diagnoses include:

- malignant melanoma
- glomus tumour
- pyogenic granuloma
- sarcoids.

Treatment

- In the elderly if slow-growing no treatment option
- Local treatment for single or few lesions may include:
  - surgical removal
  - cryotherapy
  - laser
  - radiation
  - intra-lesional cytotoxic therapy
  - aggressive systemic therapies with single or multi-agent drugs may be necessary
  - Kaposi's sarcoma due to immunosuppression or drugs may resolve if withdrawn
  - Kaposi's sarcoma associated with AIDS/HIV, control of superinfection is worthwhile as is treatment of the HIV.

Fibrous tumours

Acquired fibrokeratoma

There is a group of fibrous lesions occurring on the distal extremities which have been reclassified and renamed over the years, resulting in a number of different names:

- acquired digital fibrokeratoses
- acral fibromatosis
- periungual fibromatas
- garlic clove tumours
- acquired fibrokeratoma.

Aetiology

Trauma is suggested as a cause.

Clinical features

- Common on the digits, often near the joint with the periungual area being very common
- Slow growth rate
- Flesh-coloured or slightly translucent
- They are usually projections slightly narrower at the base, widening out and then coming to a rather pointed end
- A hyperkeratotic tip with a reddish base
- A hyperkeratotic collarette may be seen

- Lesions around the nails commonly cause a groove or sulcus on the nail plate.

  Differential diagnoses include:
- a supernumerary digit
- dermatofibroma
- osteoma
- pyogenic granuloma.

Treatment

Surgical excision.

Koenen's tumours

Periungual fibromas form one part of the condition now known as the tuberous sclerosis complex (synonyms: epiloia; Bourneville disease). There are many features which can be grouped into cutaneous, mental retardation and epilepsy. Skin problems include facial angiofibromas (adenoma sebaceum), pigmented leathery lesions (shagreen patches), hypopigmented areas (ash-leaf white macules) and Koenen's tumours. Infinite degrees of severity of the condition occur and the Koenen's tumours may be the only manifestation at times.

Dermatofibroma

Synonyms: histiocytoma cutis, fibrous histiocytoma, and sclerosing haemangioma. A dermatofibroma is a very common benign fibrous tumour, usually occurring on the extremities.

Aetiology

- Minor trauma
- Insect bites.

Clinical features

- Dermatofibroma can occur anywhere on the skin, but the limbs are the usual site.
- They may be flat or, more often, slightly protuberant.
- Usually slow-growing and less than 1 cm in diameter, they can, on occasion, be giant and over 3 cm.
- They are usually flesh coloured, but can have a yellowish tinge, mimicking xanthomata.
- At times they are slightly pigmented.
- They may have a ring of enhanced pigmentation, probably in the nature of post inflammatory hyper pigmentation.
- On palpation, they are firm to hard, with the hardness extending beyond the visual lesion. In other words, the part seen is rather like the tip of an iceberg.
- Normally they remain static for years, but some can become atrophic.
- Multiple lesions on the palms and soles have been described.

Treatment

Treatment is not required. If there is diagnostic doubt they should be biopsied or removed. Removal for this, cosmetic or pressure effect reasons must be complete or regrowth occurs.

Adnexal tumours

Eccrine poroma

This is a benign tumour of the epidermal portion of the eccrine sweat glands.

Clinical features

- The eccrine poroma is a relatively common tumour
- Occurs at any age, although usually over 40 years
- Affects both sexes
- More than a half are found in the sole or plantar surface of the toes
- Usually appears as a solitary non-tender, slightly red nodule
- May protrude or be pedunculated
- The surface may be warty or ulcerated and bleeding.

Differential diagnosis

- The common benign form should be easy to diagnose but may be confused with:
  - verrucae plantaris
  - fibromas
  - amelanotic melanoma
  - basal cell carcinoma
  - squamous cell carcinoma.

Treatment

In the benign form, surgical excision with an adequate margin is the preferred option. If the lesion is symptomless, the patient frail or the site surgically difficult, treatment need not be insisted upon if the tumour is benign.

Subungual exostosis

This lesion is a benign bony outgrowth from a terminal phalanx.

Aetiology

A history of trauma may or may not be obtained.

Clinical features

- Females are affected twice as often as males
- Usually affects the hallux
- Arises from the dorsal aspect of the terminal phalanx and appears under the distal edge of the nail plate, which it elevates but does not distort
- There may be pain from pressure
- Hard on palpation
- X-ray of the affected digit should be diagnostic. Should include antero-posterior and lateral views
- In the early stages it may be cartilaginous, non-ossified and thus radiotranslucent.

Treatment

Surgical removal is usually permanently curative.

Myxoid cyst

Synonyms: mucoid cyst or pseudocyst. These are lesions usually occurring around the distal aspect of a digit. They are very much more common on the fingers than on the toes.

Aetiology

Myxoid cysts tend to be associated with degenerative joint disease. Thus, Heberden's nodes are commonly seen in association. A tiny threadlike channel connects the cyst to the joint space.

Clinical features

- The lesions appear usually on the skin covering the terminal phalanx
- Toes can be affected, although much less commonly than the fingers
- Commonest site is near the proximal nail folds
- A small, translucent nodule appears
- Discharge may occur either spontaneously or after trauma producing a rather sticky fluid
- Depending on site they may transilluminate
- Ultrasound or magnetic resonance induction may help to resolve any diagnostic doubt.

Histology

This shows a pseudocyst with a vague capsule. Within this, there are myxomatous changes.

Treatment

- Radical excision necessitates the identification of the connection to the joint
- Cryotherapy
- Infra-red coagulation
- Multiple needling.

Ganglia

A ganglion is a cystic swelling commonly formed near the wrist. They also occur on the feet. There is dispute as to whether they are a degenerative process or a benign tumour of the tendon sheath or joint capsule.

Clinical features

On the foot, these are usually on the dorsum. In general, ganglia appear in early adult life. They may be symptomless or cause problems due to pressure. If a nerve is compressed, neurological symptoms may ensue.

Treatment

Benign and symptomless lesions may be left. They may disappear spontaneously or after a blow which ruptures them. If nerve damage or pressure effects are problems, excision may be needed. Surgery can be difficult and recurrences occur.

Piezogenic pedal papules

These lesions are generally small papular lesions on the heel provoked by pressure of standing. They can be painful.

Clinical features

The flesh-coloured nodules appear on the heels on weight bearing and disappear when the pressure is removed. Usually they occur on the medial aspect of the heel but can affect the lateral aspect.

Treatment

Usually none is very feasible. Supportive heel pads may alleviate pain.

Neurofibromatosis

Synonym: von Recklinghausen's neurofibromatosis. Neurofibromatosis is one of a mixed group of conditions affecting the skin and nerves – the neurocutaneous disorders. Since von Recklinghausen's original description, the condition has been split, mainly into neurofibromatosis 1 and neurofibromatosis 2, although other numbers are being added. The main skin involvement is in neurofibromatosis 1.

Clinical features

- Neurofibromatosis 1 is an autosomal dominant familial condition
- It occurs in about 1 : 4000 persons
- In neurofibromatosis 1 many systems can be affected. The skin changes can be divided into pigmentary and tumour ones
- Pigmentary changes start in childhood as smooth patches like milky coffee (café au lait)
- Smaller similar lesions resembling freckles aggregate in the axillae or groin
- Larger nodular or diffuse plexiform neurofibromas can be present. Can affect any area, including the foot
- Neurofibromatosis 2 is the other main variant, but is much rarer, affecting only 1 : 40 000. Skin lesions are rarer, but do include café au lait spots and tumours.

Treatment

- Monitoring and genetic counselling form much of the management
- Small numbers of neurofibromas may be amenable to surgical removal procedures for cosmetic reasons
- Some cutaneous or visceral ones may need surgery due to pressure effects or suspicion of malignant transformation.

FUNGAL INFECTIONS OF THE FEET AND NAILS

Fungal infections are the most common dermatoses of the feet. About 20% of the population are likely to be affected at some time or other during their lives. They exist as either parasites or saprophytes which, respectively, depend upon living or dead organic material for nutrition. The majority of fungi are moulds, which are composed of a network of branching filaments and look rather like cotton wool in culture. Yeasts exist as single cells and their colonies are smooth-surfaced on culture.

Dermatophyte infection

Three varieties of dermatophyte are common pathogens of the feet:

- trichophyton rubrum the commonest pathogen seen in chronic infection. Causes over 80% of all nail infections
- trichophyton mentagrophytes causes many acute infections
- tichophyton interdigitalae causes many acute infections
- epidermophyton floccosum produces a brisk inflammatory response and may, therefore, be self-resolving.

  Dermatophytes cause athlete's foot, or tinea pedis:

- about 15% of the population is affected
- prevalence rises to 25% or more in sportsmen who regularly use communal bathing facilities
- nearly always becomes established in the 4th toe cleft first
- disease can spread to all other toe clefts and onto the soles and sides of the feet and sometimes onto the dorsum of the foot
- infection – of usually one hand – is often seen, although hand infection is much less usual than foot infection
- punctate infection of the sole can occur.

Clinical types

- Toe cleft infection:
  - maceration of the skin
  - development of a single central fissure
  - can be asymptomatic
  - may produce itching and burning in the toe cleft
  - may remain confined to the 4th toe cleft almost indefinitely or can spread to other clefts
  - secondary yeast or bacterial infection is common
- Moccasin tinea pedis:
  - affects sole and sides of the foot
  - usually takes the form of a dry-type dermatitis reaction
  - scaling is often more pronounced than inflammation
  - early stages seen only in the region of the toe clefts as spread is relatively slow
  - a vesicopustular reaction can take place on the soles
  - often bilateral a unilateral picture is more suspicious of a fungal infection
  - in advanced cases the dorsum of the foot is involved
  - in such cases classic anular lesions with raised scaly edges and healing centres – ringworm
  - allergic reactions or if reactions may occur.

Differential diagnosis

- Bacterial infection alone is an unusual reaction in the toe clefts but may occur with some Gram-negative bacteria
- Psoriasis
- Pustular psoriasis
- Dermatitis
- Plantar keratodermas
- Pitted keratolysis.

Nail infection

Fungal nail infection may be caused by dermatophyte yeasts or non-dermato-phyte moulds. Yeasts more often affect fingernails. Fungal nail infection is a disease of insidious onset but thereafter progression is relentless and it does not resolve spontaneously.

There are various published clinical classifications of onychomycosis:

- distal and lateral subungual onychomycosis (DLSO)
- superficial white onychomycosis (SWO)
- proximal subungual onychomycosis (PSO)
- total dystrophic onychomycosis (TDO)
- candidal onychomycosis (CO).

Distal and lateral subungual onychomycosis (DLSO)

- Commonest variety of onychomycosis caused by dermatophytes
- Initially a disease of the hyponichium, resulting in hyperkeratosis of the distal nail bed
- Begins at the lateral edge of the nail and spreads progressively proximally down the nail
- Underside of the nail is involved causing a thick, friable and crumbly nail
- The fungus proliferates in the space between the nail plate and nail bed and this is known as a dermatophytoma
- Scytilidium dimidiatum produces a similar appearance with a black discoloration of the nail plate. Associated with patients or travellers from the tropics
- Scopulariopsis brevicaulis and some Aspergillus species are occasionally isolated but they are probably secondary pathogens to previously damaged nail
- Most non-dermatophyte moulds are resistant to antifungal drugs and nail removal is usually necessary as treatment.

Superficial white onychomycosis (SWO)

- A less common variety and is usually the result of a T. mentagrophytes infection
- Affects the dorsal surface of the nail and thus sometimes responds to topical treatment
- A dense white appearance occurs in patients with AIDS. Although this is not a true SWO, in that the whole thickness of the nail plate is involved, it is certainly white in appearance and is appropriately classified here for the sake of clinical convenience.

Proximal subungual onychomycosis (PSO)

- Yeast infection is the commonest cause of a proximal nail infection but that is dealt with under the heading of Candidal onychomycosis (CO)
- T. rubrum occasionally causes PSO where the disease begins at the proximal end of the nail
- Seen in patients with intercurrent disease such as AIDS and peripheral vascular disease.

Total dystrophic onychomycosis (TDO)

All of the above varieties will eventually produce total dystrophy of the nail which is really a classification for end-stage infection.

Candida onychomycosis (CO)

- Candidal infection of the nail can exist in four forms:
  - the commonest variety is a proximal infection of the nail secondary to a chronic paronychia. Seen in patients with wet occupations where the cuticle becomes detached from the nail plate and infection occurs in the subcuticular space
  - distal infection with yeasts is almost exclusively seen in patients with Raynaud's phenomenon
  - chronic mucocutaneous candidosis. In the most severe types there is gross thickening and hyperkeratosis of the whole nail which is packed with yeasts. Such patients are usually children who often do not survive into adult life because of the degree of immunodeficiency
  - the fourth variety of yeast infection is purely secondary to intercurrent disease and psoriatic nails are often colonised by yeasts but treatment of the yeast will rarely significantly improve the clinical appearance because psoriasis is the primary defect.

Tinea incognito

It is appropriate to mention this variety of fungal infection, although it is a poor name which legitimises misdiagnosed and mistreated fungal infection with topical steroids. It can be seen on the feet and lower legs when fungal infection is mistaken for a dermatitis reaction and treated with topical steroids. If there is clinical doubt and treatment must be instituted then it is always safer to begin with a topical antifungal which will do no harm to dermatitis, whereas a topical steroid will enhance a fungal infection.

Laboratory diagnosis

- In cases of skin infection a skin scraping should be taken from the edge of the lesion which can either be done dry or following dampening of the area with saline.
- Because nail infection is primarily a disease of the nail bed rather than the nail plate, collection of hyperkeratotic material from beneath the nail is always best and, of course, a specimen from the most proximal part of the infection contains the most active fungus.
- Nail clippings are less likely to yield fungus and are more difficult to handle in a laboratory.
- Scrapings from the nail surface are of no use at all in cases other than SWO.
- Direct microscopy is entirely adequate for diagnosis of infection and institution of treatment.
- It is mandatory to confirm the diagnosis of infection in nail disease prior to commencing oral therapy.
- Although fungal nail infection is the commonest cause of nail dystrophy, it still accounts for only 50% of all cases of dystrophic nails which present and this confirms the need for accurate laboratory diagnosis.
- If the disease is strongly suspected on clinical grounds and the laboratory test is negative in microscopy and culture, then it should be repeated at least once and possibly twice before fungal infection is excluded.

Treatment of fungal foot and nail infections

- Interdigital tinea pedis is best treated topically.
- An antifungal cream should always be used. Antifungal foot powders are only useful prophylactically.
- Both azoles and allylamines inhibit sterol biosynthesis in the fungal cell wall.
- Topical allylamines are the treatment of choice in interdigital foot infection and topical terbinafine is now available over the counter in both regular and 'once-only' formulations. Although more costly than topical azoles, its higher cure rates over shorter treatment duration together with its lower relapse rates make it a much more attractive option.
- Compliance is a problem with longer treatments and compliance with the full course of therapy using azole drugs is much less likely.
- Systemic treatment will be required in some cases for infection of the palms and soles where the keratin is much thicker and there may be difficulty in penetration of topical agents.
- Creams have no part to play in the treatment of nail infection and nail lacquers are generally ineffective other than in the case of superficial white onychomycosis.
- There are no topical allylamine preparations designed specifically for nails and amorolfine nail lacquer (Loceryl), which is probably the most effective agent, should only be recommended for SWO or possibly as an adjunct to systemic therapy.
- Oral agents are the best treatment option for onychomycosis:
  - griseofulvin is a weakly fungistatic antidermatophyte agent. It remains the only drug licensed for use in children
  - ketoconazole is no longer licensed for use in skin and nail infections because of hepatotoxicity
  - itraconazole is a leading player in the treatment of foot and nail infection and is given in nail infections in a pulsed fashion; 400 mg per day of the drug is given for 1 week per month and repeated three or four times
  - terbinafine is a leading player in the treatment of foot and nail infection, is the most potent antidermatophyte agent and is given in a dose of 250 mg daily for 6 weeks in fingernails and for 3 months in toenails
  - fluconazole is a useful drug in yeast infections but it has relatively weak antidermatophyte activity.
- Side effects of oral treatments include the following:
  - itraconazole and terbinafine have some potential side effects. Minor side effects such as nausea and itch are seen in only about 5% of cases.
  - terbinafine does cause taste disturbance in about 1 : 400.
  - hepatotoxicity occurs in about 1 : 50 000 cases in terbinafine-treated patients.
  - itraconazole causes abnormality of liver enzymes somewhat more frequently but patients rarely become symptomatic.

Although the incidence of significant side effects with systemic antifungal agents compares favourably with many other drugs, there is no doubt that there is some resistance on the part of both patients and medical attendants to their prescription in nail infection. Topical agents, which are largely ineffective, continue to maintain a significant market share and ongoing development of effective topical agents for nail infections remains a priority.

Following successful treatment of systemic infection prophylactic measures should be taken to prevent re-infection:

- nail infection is secondary to toe cleft disease and any evidence of recurrence of toe-cleft infection should be treated enthusiastically.
- prevention of toe-cleft infection is possible with antifungal foot powders or the wearing of small plastic socks while swimming.
- the former is probably a more feasible option and any antifungal foot powder should be applied after swimming or using communal bathing places.
- particular attention must be paid to the toe clefts and such use of powder has been shown to be useful in preventing re-infection in regular users.
- the degree of spread via contaminated footwear is unknown, but it is theoretically possible and powder may be applied to the inside of shoes as well.

Chapter | **4** |

General foot disorders

Introduction and terminology

Clinical biomechanical analysis of foot and leg function is essentially qualitative and is an exercise in observation and examination:

- observation and quantification of joint position
- examination of the quality, range and direction of motion of the joints
- observation, quantification and examination of the functioning limb in gait
- advances in technology impact on orthosis therapy prescription, provision and evaluation.

The neutral position of the joints of the lower limb are used as a reference point

Hip joint neutral:

- leg is in line with the trunk in the sagittal plane
- femoral condyles lie in the frontal plane
- legs are parallel to one another
- feet slightly apart and abducted (from this position the hip joint can flex, extend, adduct, abduct, rotate and circumduct).

Knee joint neutral:

- joint fully extended
- thigh and lower leg in line (from this position the knee joint can only flex).

Ankle joint neutral:

- foot lies on a flat horizontal weight-bearing surface
- leg is perpendicular (from this position, the ankle joint may dorsiflex and plantarflex).

Subtalar joint in or near its hypothetical neutral position:

- posterior aspect of the calcaneus perpendicular to the weight-bearing surface (from this position the subtalar joint may supinate and pronate).

Midtarsal joint (MTJ) complex neutral:

- all metatarsal heads lie on the horizontal weight-bearing surface
- joint maximally pronated (from this position the MTJ complex will only supinate).

1st metatarsophalangeal joint neutral:

- plantar aspect of the hallux and the 1st MTPJ in ground contact
- hallux neither adducted nor abducted (from this position the 1st metatarsophalangeal joint (MTPJ) may dorsiflex, plantarflex, adduct, abduct and circumduct).

1st ray neutral:

- 1st metatarsal head in line with the lesser metatarsal heads
- metatarsal heads lie parallel to the ground (from this position the first ray can dorsiflex and invert, and plantarflex and evert).

Lesser rays neutral:

- they are most dorsiflexed and lying parallel to the weight-bearing surface (from this position the lesser rays will only plantarflex).

5th ray neutral:

- parallel to the weight-bearing surface and inline with the other metatarsal heads

The principle of compensation

Compensation occurs when a joint cannot function maximally and adjacent joint function is modified to normalise foot function.

Joint motion is classed as sub-maximal if the total range of motion of the joint is:

- too great
- too little
- in the wrong direction
- of poor quality.

Joint position is abnormal if the adjacent bones and body segments are:

- malformed
- damaged due to trauma or disease
- misaligned.

There are a number of abnormalities or variations from the norm that result in abnormal foot and leg function. The common causative abnormalities are outlined below.

The gait or walking cycle

The gait or walking cycle is the sequence of events in one limb during one complete stride. The cycle is divided into:

- stance phase
- swing phase.

Stance phase is subdivided into three periods:

- the contact period – foot and limb should be unlocked and mobile
- the midstance period – converting from one state to the other
- the propulsive period – a rigid and stable lever.

Occurrence:

- the stance phase of gait occurs from heel strike to foot
- midstance period of the stance phase of gait occurs from foot flat to heel lift
- propulsive period of the stance phase of gait occurs from heel lift to toe off.

FRONTAL PLANE ANOMALIES OR MALALIGNMENTS OF THE REARFOOT

The inverted or varus rearfoot

Rearfoot varus

Rearfoot varus is a congenital structural abnormality of the rearfoot which is inverted to the weight-bearing surface; the subtalar joint is in neutral position and the mid-tarsal joint is maximally pronated around both axes.

Causes

- Result of a congenital varus (frontal plane) abnormality of the leg or foot
- Fractures
- Other severe trauma, particularly to growing bones
- As a result of subjects displaying genu vara (bow legs)
- Tibia vara (bowing of the lower third of the tibia)
- Tibial epiphyseal vara (varus abnormality of the tibial epiphysis)
- Varus deformity arises as a frontal plane anomaly of the talus (talar vara)
- Calcaneus (calcaneal vara)
- Subtalar joint (subtalar vara).

Compensatory mechanisms

The normal foot will present to the ground (at initial contact) in a slightly inverted position. In rearfoot varus the foot is in a more inverted position at the start of the contact period. Additional subtalar joint (STJ) pronation is termed 'compensation', and is abnormal and excessive.

Excessive pronation at the STJ:

- increases the range of motion of the forefoot on the rearfoot at the MTJ
- loads the medial side of the foot during the midstance period
- results in the ground reactive force (GRF) causing supination of the MTJ
- means that the foot is unlocked and hypermobile
- may mean that the foot will rapidly supinate and recover some or all of its stability before toe-off
- is compensated for by plantar flexion of the 1st metatarsal
- results is gait modification – abductory twist.

Classifications

- Fully compensated
- Uncompensated – no additional STJ pronation available
- Partially compensated.

The signs and symptoms of an uncompensated rearfoot varus include the following:

- hyperkeratotic skin lesions along the lateral side of the foot
- loss of foot mobility
- tailor's bunion
- pressure symptoms and hyperkeratotic lesions under the 1st metatarsal head
- repeated lateral ankle sprains may occur
- symptoms resulting from disordered shock attenuation
- symptoms resulting from disordered transverse plane motion of the limb.

The signs and symptoms of a fully compensated rearfoot varus include the following:

- Excessive pronation at the STJ
- lowering of medial 'arch' height
- haglund's deformity
- reduced 1st MTPJ motion
- tailor's bunion deformity
- re-supinator muscles may become fatigued and traumatised – presenting clinically as anterior or posterior 'shin splints'
- low back pain
- repeated lateral ankle sprains are common.

The signs and symptoms of partially compensated rearfoot varus varies with the compensation available at STJ and reflects aspects of compensated and uncompensated rearfoot varus.

Treatment

Compensated rearfoot varus:

- short-term: symptomatic treatment includes the use of clinical padding, strapping and physical therapies
- long-term: to negate compensatory pronation at the STJ with functional foot orthoses with intrinsic or extrinsic medial posting.

Uncompensated rearfoot varus:

- accommodative orthoses which off-load and protect traumatised areas
- shoe advice.

The everted or valgus rearfoot

A true rearfoot valgus is a rare primary congenital osseous abnormality, presenting as a structural abnormality in which the rearfoot is everted relative to the weight-bearing surface when the STJ is in its neutral position and the MTJ is maximally pronated around both axes.

A Valgus rearfoot is more commonly a secondary abnormality and appears mostly as compensation for a primary abnormality elsewhere in the limb or foot such as:

- forefoot varus
- forefoot supinatus
- mobile forefoot valgus
- genu valgum
- trauma, such as a Pott's or bimalleolar fracture
- agenesis of the distal aspect of the fibula
- congenital absence of a fibula
- rupture of tibialis posterior tendon
- rheumatoid disease

- tarsal coalition
- Charcot's neuroarthropathy
- footballer's ankle.

FRONTAL PLANE ANOMALIES OR MALALIGNMENTS OF THE FOREFOOT

The inverted or varus forefoot

True rearfoot varus

Forefoot varus is a congenital osseous structural deformity in which the plantar plane of the forefoot is inverted relative to the plantar plane of the rearfoot when the STJ is in its neutral position and the MTJ is maximally pronated around both its axes.

Causes

Forefoot varus is assumed to be an inherited structural condition due to a reduction in the developmental valgus rotation of the head and neck of the talus.

Classifications

Forefoot varus is classified according to the amount of compensatory STJ pronation available:

- fully compensated
- uncompensated – no available compensatory STJ pronation
- partially-compensated – some available STJ pronation.

Compensatory mechanisms

In the normal foot, at the midpoint of midstance, the calcaneus is vertical with STJ near its neutral position, MTJ is maximally pronated about both its axes and the plantar planes of the forefoot and rearfoot are parallel to one another and to the ground.

In an uncompensated forefoot varus, at the midpoint of midstance:

- the plantar plane of the forefoot is inverted relative to the plantar plane of the rearfoot
- the calcaneus is vertical, the STJ is in neutral and the MTJ is maximally pronated
- the foot weight bears normally until after the 5th metatarsal head contacts the ground
- the forefoot is inverted to allow the medial side of the forefoot to contact the ground
- the fore foot compensates by everting or pronating excessively to allow the medial side of the forefoot to contact the ground
- excessive pronation at the forefoot is not possible
- weight bearing occurs on the heel and lateral side of the forefoot only
- the foot abducts by using the 5th metatarsal head as a pivot, to load the medial side of the foot after the midpoint of midstance.

  In a fully compensated forefoot varus:

- foot contact is normal until the midpoint of midstance
- the foot continues to pronate to allow the medial area of the forefoot to bear weight

- the calcaneus everts as the STJ abnormally and excessively pronates
- the plantar plane of the forefoot is inverted relative to the plantar plane of the rearfoot, but it is weight bearing and is parallel to the ground
- the MTJ is unlocked
- the forefoot is hypermobile.

A partially compensated forefoot varus is one in which there is some compensatory pronation available at the STJ, but insufficient to allow the forefoot to evert completely onto the weight-bearing surface.

The signs and symptoms of a fully compensated forefoot varus include:

- calcaneal eversion in static stance and during gait from midstance to toe-off
- abduction of forefoot on rearfoot
- excessive lowering of the medial 'arch' on weight bearing
- forefoot deformities – hallux abductovalgus, lesser toe deformities, associated hyperkeratotic skin lesions and other soft-tissue pathologies
- plantar fasciitis
- plantar digital neuritis
- non-specific 'arch' strains
- ankle tendonopathies
- thigh, groin, shin and knee problems together with disordered postural stability
- low back pain.

The signs and symptoms of an uncompensated forefoot varus include:

- relatively joint immobility
- poor shock-absorption qualities
- it is often seen in conjunction with a rearfoot varus.
- calcaneus remains vertical at the end of the contact period
- excessive lateral weight bearing during stance
- abductory twist of the foot
- heel adducts towards the midline of the body
- hyperkeratotic lesions over the plantar surface of the interphalangeal joint (IPJ) of the hallux
- knee problems
- compensatory plantarflexion of the 1st metatarsal.

The signs and symptoms of partially compensated forefoot varus show a mix of the features of both fully and uncompensated forefoot varus, depending on the degree of compensation, and where it takes place.

Treatment

In fully compensated forefoot varus:

- orthoses are used to reduce the compensatory excessive pronation and hypermobility of the forefoot.

Uncompensated rearfoot varus requires and accommodative orthosis.

Forefoot supinatus

Forefoot supinatus is an acquired soft-tissue deformity of the longitudinal axis of the midtarsal joint where the forefoot is inverted relative to the rearfoot when the STJ is in neutral position and the MTJ is maximally pronated around both its axes.

Causes

Any abnormality which results in excessive pronation of the STJ has the potential to induce resultant eversion of the calcaneus including:

- forefoot varus
- ankle equinus
- abnormal limb position.

Clinical recognition

Forefoot supinatus has a similar appearance to a foot with forefoot varus. The two conditions are differentiated by the application of a pronatory force to the dorsum of the foot at the talonavicular joint:

- forefoot supinatus – spongy resistance to pronatory force, forefoot inversion reduces
- forefoot varus – firm resistance to pronatory force, forefoot inversion reduces if STJ is allowed to evert.

Treatment

- Control abnormal calcaneal eversion
- Forefoot supinatus should not be supported by an orthotic
- The soft-tissue supinatus contracture of the forefoot should be totally or partially reduced when taking the plaster impression of the forefoot
- An orthosis should be manufactured to reflect this degree of control of the calcaneal.

The everted or valgus forefoot

Forefoot valgus

Forefoot valgus is a congenital osseous deformity where the plantar plane of the forefoot is everted relative to the plantar plane of the rearfoot when the STJ is in the neutral position and the MTJ is maximally pronated around both its axes.

Causes

- Head and neck of the talus undergoes a valgus rotation on the body of the talus during normal development
- In forefoot valgus an excessive amount of developmental valgus rotation results in the plantar plane of the forefoot being everted relative to the hindfoot
- If the 1st metatarsal head lies on a lower plane than the lesser metatarsal heads this is a plantarflexed first ray (i.e. partial forefoot valgus)
- A plantarflexed first ray is an acquired condition resulting from a muscular imbalance.

Classifications

- Total forefoot valgus
- Partial forefoot valgus due to plantarflexion of the first ray
- Rigid-type forefoot valgus
- Mobile-type forefoot valgus.

    In total forefoot valgus:

- the plantar plane of the forefoot is everted relative to the plantar plane of the rearfoot. The metatarsal heads are in line one with the other but are everted relative to the rearfoot.

In partial forefoot valgus:

- the first ray is plantarflexed in relation to the lesser metatarsal heads which lie on the same plane as the rearfoot.

Rigid-type forefoot valgus

- Rigid forefoot valgus is immobile
- The rearfoot is in a normal relationship to the lower leg
- The 1st metatarsal head will contact the ground before the 5th
- Forefoot loads from medial to lateral
- GRF attempts to supinate the forefoot about the longitudinal axis of the MTJ
- MTJ cannot compensate adequately for the forefoot eversion, additional compensatory supination is required at the STJ
- Leg is externally rotated with lateral instability of the ankle/ST joint and the knees.

The signs and symptoms of rigid forefoot valgus:

- a high-arched 'pes cavus'-type foot
- MTJ shows reduced mobility
- lesser toes retracted or clawed
- hyperkeratotic pressure lesions on plantar aspects of the 1st and 5th metatarsal heads
- posterolateral calcaneal irritation (development of Haglund's deformity)
- difficulties in obtaining suitable footwear because of high arch and the deformed lesser toes
- excessive lateral shoe sole wear.

Mobile-type forefoot valgus

- Heel contact is normal
- Forefoot loads under the MTPJs in the order one to five
- Foot is characteristically mobile and distorts under load
- 1st ray dorsiflexes and the MTPJ supinates (unlocks) and resultant forefoot mobility.

Signs and symptoms of mobile forefoot valgus:

- forefoot instability results in hallux abducto valgus (HAV) due to forefoot instabiligy
- lesser toe deformities
- plantar hyperkeratosis under the central metatarsal heads
- 5th toe corns and a tendency to splayed forefoot and Tailor's bunion
- plantar fasciitis
- plantar digital neuritis
- medial sesamoiditis
- 1st metatarsal-cuneiform joint exostosis

Treatment

All presentations of forefoot valgus respond to the following:

- Orthotic therapy to accommodate the everted position of the forefoot
- accommodation of the plantarflexed position of the 1st metatarsal head in partial forefoot valgus

- orthoses that projectdistal to the metatarsal heads
- orthoses to reduce 1st ray dorsiflexion and MTPJ supination (For mobile forefoot valgus).

OTHER FRONTAL PLANE ANOMALIES AFFECTING FOOT FUNCTION

Leg-length discrepancy

The effect of leg-length discrepancy (LLD) on the foot and leg disrupts the normal pain-free function of the lumbar spine, the limb and the foot.

Causes

- Idiopathic unequal development
- Unilateral coxa vara
- Pelvic abnormalities
- Fractures or surgery resulting in shortening of the limb
- Surgery or pathology resulting in limb overgrowth
- Several diseases and abnormalities.

Effects

- Altered gait patterns
- Equinus contracture at the ankle
- Increased energy expenditure in gait
- Runners with LLD tend to present with:
  - increased vertebral disc, low-back symptoms
  - increased incidence of tibial stress fractures
  - knee pain
  - shin splints
  - painful heel syndrome
  - symptomatic hallux valgus
  - sciatica
- Increased activity of the lumbar spine muscles
- Pain in the lumbar spine
- Increased tensile stress at the short leg side
- Increased compressive stress at the long leg side
- Intravertebral disc becomes wedge-shaped
- Weight shift to longer leg
- Lowering of the shoulder on the long side
- Asymmetrical pronation
- LLD >2 cm predisposes to early heel lift/ankle equinus on the shorter leg
- Increased pelvic tilt and asymmetrical pelvic rotation
- Shoulder tilt
- Scoliosis of the spine
- Increased mechanical stress on the hip joint of the longer limb
- Knee pathologies.

Symptoms

- Arthritis of the knee
- Psoasitis

- Anterior knee pain
- Shin splints
- Metatarsalgia
- Sacroiliitis
- Achilles tendonitis
- Quadriceps strain
- Pes anserinus bursitis
- Groin strain
- Peroneal tendonitis
- Neck pain
- Intermetatarsal neuroma
- Osteitis pubis
- Sesamoiditis
- Sinus tarsi syndrome
- Limp.

Management

LLD is managed by applying height correction to the short limb and the use of orthoses to control excessive foot pronation in the long limb:

- a simple heel lift incorporated into a functional foot orthoses
- in LLD >2 cm the use of heel lift is contraindicated. A full-length sole lift, with or without an in-shoe orthotic.

SAGITTAL PLANE ANOMALIES OR MALALIGNMENTS

Ankle equinus

A congenital or acquired functional deficiency of sagittal plane motion at the ankle joint where there is limited dorsiflexion of the ankle joint when the STJ is in the neutral position.

Aetiology and presentations

A range of foot and limb conditions are characterised by ankle equinus. These include:

- congenital or acquired contraction of the Achilles tendon complex
- apparent or pseudo ankle equinus in cases where there is a plantarflexed or equinus forefoot
- an equinus gait due to talipes, spasticity or other neurological disorders
- unilateral equinus deformity of the shorter limb as a compensation for limb length
- excessive use of high-heeled shoes.

Classification

Ankle equinus, as other functional abnormalities of the foot, is classified by the degree of compensation:

- fully compensated ankle equinus occurs if the foot achieves 10° dorsiflexion at the ankle joint
- uncompensated ankle equinus occurs if 10° of dorsiflexion cannot be achieved
- partially compensated ankle equinus occurs if all available ankle joint dorsiflexion plus abnormal and excessive subtalar joint pronation is insufficient to achieve 10° of dorsiflexion and allow normal limb movement during midstance.

Compensation for reduced dorsiflexion at the ankle joint may occur in the lower leg:

- premature heel lift
- genu recurvatum
- excessive knee flexion
- an abductory twist.

Treatment

- A full biomechanical evaluation to establish the cause
- Treatments include:
  - posterior muscle-group stretching regimens
  - orthoses therapy and footwear advice.

Functional hallux limitus

Functional hallux limitus occurs when there is sufficient dorsiflexion of the hallux at the 1st MTPJ when tested in the non-weight-bearing foot, but insufficient dorsiflexion of the hallux at the 1st MTPJ to allow normal gait when tested in the weight-bearing foot.

Sagittal plane blockade

A foot with functional hallux limitus shows blockade of sagittal plane motion of the hallux at the first MTPJ until the positional abnormality that caused the limitation no longer influences the movement of the hallux.

Hypermobile medial column/first ray

A hypermobile 1st ray is a foot in which the 1st ray is less stable than in the normal foot.

ABNORMALITIES OF ARCH HEIGHT

Encompasses pes planus and pes cavus.

- Pes planus describes a foot with a low medial profile due to:
  - overpronation at the subtalar joint
  - a hyperflexible
  - a foot damaged by trauma or disease
- Pes cavus describes a foot that has an abnormally high medially arched profile due to:
  - abnormal development
  - neurological disease
  - congenital foot abnormality
  - trauma.

Pes planus

Pes planus can be subdivided into rigid or flexible pes planus:

- functional pes planus – overpronation of the STJ
- congenital rigid flat foot
- congenital flexible flat foot

- acquired rigid flat foot
- neurological flat feet – rigid or flexible flat foot as sequelae to poliomyelitis, cerebral palsy, peripheral nerve injuries and muscular dystrophy.

Consequences

Flexible flat foot causes include:

- postural symptoms involving the lower limb, pelvis and spine
- apropulsive gait
- forefoot disruption
- foot pathologies.

Treatment

- Identification of underlying cause
- Severe flat feet, involving late-stage tibialis posterior dysfunction and flat foot of congenital or traumatic origin respond poorly to conservative treatments
- Refer for an orthopaedic or podiatric surgery opinion
- Rigid flat foot causes a range of symptoms – treatment is palliative, maximising available function
- Refer for surgery.

Pes cavus

A pes cavus foot also shows the following characteristics:

- limited or absent STJ range of motion
- all foot joints show reduced range of motion
- altered angles of inclination of the foot bones
- retraction of the toes including the hallux (trigger toe)
- inversion of the rearfoot
- abnormal plantar weight distribution
- decreased or absent ankle joint dorsiflexion
- apropulsive gait
- neuromuscular, congenital or familial aetiology.

Aetiology

- Neuromuscular dysfunction that results in spasm of peroneus longus or tibialis posterior or weakness of peroneus longus and brevis. Associated with poliomyelitis, cerebral palsy, spina bifida, hereditary motor and sensory neuropathies, Friedreich's ataxia and spinal cord tumours
- Severe metatarsus adductus
- Talipes equinovarus deformities.

Presentations of highly arched feet not in association with neuromuscular dysfunction, congenital abnormality or familial predisposition include:

- rigid plantarflexed 1st ray
- rigid forefoot valgus
- uncompensated or partially compensated rearfoot varus
- limb-length inequality where the foot of the shorter leg supinates
- pseudo ankle equinus.

DISORDERS OF THE FOOT

Osteochondrosis/osteochondritis

Osteochondrosis is the generic term for a group of syndromes sharing the common pathology of idiopathic bone disease characterised by:

- interruption of normal enchondral ossification
- focal death of the local trabeculated bone
- onset during childhood
- focal bone deformation during the healing phase
- altered shape of the involved bone sites causes pathologies later in life.

Classification

Osteochondritis – classification in relation to the anatomical location of the enchondral ossification defect:

- osteochondritis of the *primary articular epiphysis* – e.g. Freiberg's disease and Kohler's disease
- osteochondritis of the *secondary articular epiphysis* – e.g. osteochondritis dissicans of the talus
- osteochondritis of the *non-articular epiphysis* – e.g. Sever's disease and Iselin's disease.

Osteochondritis – classification in relation to effects caused by local forces on the area of diseased enchondral bone:

- crushing apophysitis
- traction apophysitis
- fragmentation osteochondritis.

Aetiology

The aetiology of the various presentations of osteochondritis is unknown but is linked to:

- hereditary factors
- local trauma
- nutritional factors
- local ischaemia within the affected area of bone.

Diagnosis

- Plain radiographs usually used for diagnosis
- Lesions identified using bone scan
- Computerised axial tomography (CAT) scan
- Magnetic resonance imaging (MRI).

Differential diagnosis

The differential diagnosis for all of the osteochondritides includes:

- osteomyelitis
- bone tumours
- fractures.

Treatment

The treatment of all presentations of osteochondritis focuses on:

- rest
- immobilisation
- use of pain-killers
- early initiation of treatment, which is especially important
- a period of rehabilitation and exercise, which is required following prolonged rest:
  - assists in a return to normal muscular function
  - helps to overcome disuse atrophy of limb muscles
- in-shoe orthosis to reduce weight-bearing at an affected metatarsophalangeal joint
- possible surgical excision of bone fragments within the joint capsule.

Presentations of osteochondritis within the foot

Freiberg's disease (infraction)

The disease affects the metatarsal head(s) and patients are normally female and aged between 12 and 15 years.

Pathology

- Presents unilaterally or bilaterally
- Head of the 2nd metatarsal affected in 70% of cases
- The 3rd metatarsal head affected in 30% of cases
- Due to local trauma during the gait cycle, especially toe-off
- The blood supply to the epiphyseal plate is interrupted causing avascular necrosis within the metatarsal head.

Clinical picture

The patient presents with:

- pain
- swelling
- bruising on the dorsum of the foot
- a limp
- worsening pain on weight bearing and activity
- decreased range of motion at affected MTPJ
- pain and crepitus on passive movement.

Diagnosis and differential diagnosis

- Early stages of the disease: plain radiographs may show little apparent bone involvement
- Later stages: plain radiographs may show new bone growth in the affected area.

The differential diagnoses:

- march fracture
- rheumatoid arthritis
- intermetatarsal bursitis
- overuse injuries in relation to sports or dancing.

Kohler's disease

This disease affects the ossification centre of the navicular in young boys aged between 2 and 9 years.

Pathology

- Repetitive minor trauma to the navicular.

Clinical picture

The patient presents with:
- pain
- swelling
- focal tenderness.

Osteochondritis dissicans of the talus

The talar head is commonly affected or the trochlear surface may also be involved.

Pathology

The bone lesion is classified in four stages of presentation:

Stage I – Small area of trabeculated subchrondral bone becomes compressed and ischaemic

Stage II – Unsupported cortical bone begins to separate from the body of the bone

Stage III – Detached fragment dislodges

Stage IV – Detached fragment moves within the joint.

Clinical picture

- Painful, swollen ankle
- Location of the pain and the swelling:
  - osteochondritis dissicans of the talar head – pain and swelling in the medial area of the MTJ
  - osteochondritis dissicans of the trochlear surface – pain and swelling at the anterior aspect of the ankle
  - a loose body within the ankle or talonavicular joints – site of the pain and swelling is less constant.

Sever's disease

This is the most common cause of heel pain in children aged between 7 and 12 years. It is not a true avascular necrosis, but more accurately traction apophysitis.

Pathology

- Heel pain as a result of overuse

Clinical picture

The condition may:
- be unilateral or bilateral
- involve pain and tenderness at the posterior aspect of the calcaneus
- present with pain maximal after vigorous or impact exercise
- be associated with warmth and oedema at the posterior heel area
- affect boys more often than girls.

Diagnosis and differential diagnoses

- Increased pain on passive dorsiflexion of the foot
- Exacerbation of symptoms when standing on tiptoe
- Radiographs of the calcaneus are normal in the early stages of the disease
- Once the disorder progresses, apophyseal area shows sclerosis and fragmentation.

The differential diagnosis includes:

- a duck-bill fracture of the posterior leaflet of the calcaneus
- Achilles tendon pathologies
- deep retrocalcaneal bursitis.

Iselin's disease

This is a traction apophysitis that affects the base of the 5th metatarsal.

Clinical picture

- Inflammation
- Swelling and tenderness
- Bruising and pain.

Differential diagnosis

- Stress fracture of the styloid process
- Jones fracture or avulsion fracture of the styloid.

DISORDERS OF THE REARFOOT

Posterior heel pain

Superficial retrocalcaneal bursitis

Clinical features

- Usually affects adolescent females
- Pain at posterior aspect of the heel
- Inflamed, fluctuant and tender
- Palpable hypertrophy of the superficial fascia
- Underlying bone hypertrophy.

Diagnosis

- Presenting signs and symptoms
- Oblique-lateral radiographs of the rearfoot.

Differential diagnosis

- Sever's disease
- Huglund's deformity
- Deep retrocalcaneal bursitis.

Treatment

A conservative approach is indicated:

- appropriate accommodative footwear
- cooling lotions or rubefacients to reduce inflammation
- clinical padding
- plastazote heel cup

- footwear modifications
- surgery.

Deep retrocalcaneal bursitis

Clinical features

- Diffuse pain at posterior aspect of the heel
- Exacerbated by active dorsiflexion of the foot
- Local warmth and swelling
- Swelling is palapable on either side of the Achilles tendon.

Differential diagnosis

- Achilles tendonitis
- Superficial retrocalcaneal bursitis
- Rheumatoid or seronegative arthritides
- Sever's disease.

Treatment

- Rest
- Footwear review
- Simple heel raise
- Aspiration of the bursa and corticosteroid injection.

Achilles tendonitis

This is a painful debilitating inflammation of the Achilles tendon.

It is a degenerative condition which does not produce painful symptoms during activity and is characterised by a swelling or a nodule approximately 5 cm superior to the insertion of the tibialis anterior tendon.

Peritendonitis with tendonosis is characterised by local pain and swelling along the distal tendon that increases with activity and may progress to partial or complete rupture.

Clinical picture

- Pain in the distal part of the tendon
- Pain during strenuous activity that eases with rest
- Severe unrelenting pain
- Soft tissues are hot and swollen
- Associated tendonosis may be present
- Gradual onset.

Diagnosis and differential diagnosis

- Pain induced by plantarflexion of the ankle against resistance
- Severe cases show inflammation and tears in the tendon on MRI
- Radiographs show local inflammation.

  Differential diagnosis:

- Haglund's deformity
- deep retrocalcaneal bursitis
- inflammatory arthritides
- partial or total rupture of the Achilles tendon.

Treatment

- Orthotic therapy
- Stretching exercises *before* sporting activity
- Heel raise
- Advice on training and pre-stretching
- Rest from strenuous sports activity
- Footwear advice
- Physical therapies.

Rupture and partial rupture of the Achilles tendon

The tendon is prone to rupture 2–5 cm from its insertion on the posterior surface of the calcaneus.

Clinical picture

- Palpable painful swelling along the distal part of the tendon
- A discontinuity along the length of the tendon
- Inability to stand on tiptoe
- History of a severe pain and a sudden sensation of something snapping at the back of the heel.

Treatment

- Immobilisation in a below-knee cast or Aircast® boot
- Surgical repair.

Plantar heel pain

Pain of the plantar aspect of the heel may be caused by a number of pathologies:

- heel pain syndrome
- plantar fascia rupture
- fat pad atrophy
- stress fractures of the calcaneus
- proximal plantar fasciitis
- distal plantar fasciitis
- plantar fibromatosis
- tendonitis of the flexor hallucis longus tendon
- tumour of the calcaneus
- nerve entrapment
- injury.

Heel pain syndrome

This is characterised by inflammation of the proximal portion of the plantar fascia and presents in the 40–60 age group.

Clinical picture

- Gradual and increasing pain at the medial-central heel area
- Radiates into the medial longitudinal arch
- Sharp or severe pain
- Pain worse on weight bearing subsides on walking
- Recurs after periods of rest
- Tightness of the Achilles tendon
- Pain is elicited by traction to the plantar fascia.

Diagnosis and differential diagnosis

- Characteristic pattern of pain
- Diagnosis confirmed by ultrasonography and radioisotope bone scans.

  Differential diagnosis includes:

- foot strain or plantar fasciitis
- plantar calcaneal bursitis
- calcaneal fracture
- entrapment neuropathy
- seronegative inflammatory joint disease
- seropositive rheumatoid disease.

Treatment

- Sponge heel cushion
- Ring or doughnut pad
- A figure-of-eight crepe bandage
- A semi compressed felt tarsal platform
- Temporary antipronatory orthoses
- Supportive orthoses
- Dynamic therapies
- Injected hydrocortisone
- Surgery.

Tarsal tunnel syndrome

An uncommon entrapment neuropathy affecting the posterior tibial nerve.

Clinical features

- Burning pain
- Paraesthesia
- Tingling or pins and needles
- Symptoms are exacerbated by weight bearing
- Tinel's sign
- Plantar and digital sensory neuropathy with weakness of the intrinsic muscles.

Treatment

- Clinical padding
- Moulded cushioned orthoses
- Relevant drug therapies
- Surgical treatment.

Tibialis posterior tendon dysfunction

- A disabling condition arising as the direct result of the loss of function of the posterior tibial tendon.

Aetiology

The cause of tibialis posterior dysfunction is unclear but a number of factors are associated with the development of the condition, including:

- obesity
- excessive foot pronation
- structural and anatomical anomalies

- inflammatory joint diseases
- collagen vascular disease
- direct trauma
- indirect trauma
- iatrogenic events.

Pathology

Tibialis posterior dysfunction is classified into four stages:

Stage 1 – Asymptomatic stage
Stage 2 – Initial symptomatic stage
Stage 3 – Marked dysfunction stage
Stage 4 – Marked loss of foot function.

Clinical picture

- 50% have a history of local trauma
- Typically presents at stage 2 or in the sub-acute phase with:
  - diffuse swelling
  - tenderness and warmth
  - instability
- In stage 3 or the chronic phase:
  - a gradual loss of the height of the medial longitudinal arch (MLA)
  - a developing unilateral flat foot
  - lower leg fatigue
  - excessive foot abduction
  - excessive medial heel shoe wear.

Diagnosis and differential diagnosis

- Direct pressure along the course of the tendon elicits pain
- Reduced tibialis posterior muscle power on inversion of the foot
- Partial tendon rupture exhibits a distinct defect along the tendon
- Fully ruptured tendon cannot be palpated along its length
- No inversion of foot against resistance
- Partial or complete rupture is accompanied by pain at the navicular tuberosity
- MRI is the imaging modality of choice.

Differential diagnosis includes:

- bone anomalies
- fracture of the medial malleolus
- subtalar tarsal coalition
- medial sinus tarsitis
- soft-tissue anomalies
- true or apparent leg length inequality.

Treatment

- Implement rapidly and aggressively
- Non-steroidal anti-inflammatory drugs
- Ultrasound therapy
- Strap rearfoot into inversion
- Soft temporary orthoses
- Bespoke rigid antipronatory orthoses
- Plaster immobilisation of the foot in an inverted position
- Surgical intervention.

Tarsal coalition

Tarsal coalition is an autosomal dominant, congenital condition in which two or more bones in the midfoot and/or hindfoot are conjoined due to a failure of development of the intervening joint.

Clinical presentation

Presents with:

- a flat foot
- associated pain in the foot and lateral compartment of the leg
- relieved by rest, aggravated by activity
- eversion ankle sprains.

Diagnosis and differential diagnosis

- Imaging
- Plain radiographs require special views to visualise tarsal coalitions.

  Differential diagnosis includes:

- bone tumours
- rheumatological disease
- fractures about the STJ.

Treatment

The early treatment of a non-ossified tarsal coalition includes:

- immobilisation of the foot
- use of an ankle-foot orthosis or ankle calliper
- surgery.

MIDFOOT DISORDERS

Plantar fibromatosis

Fibroma or fibrous nodules develop within the plantar fascia.

Clinical features

- Single or multiple, painful or asymptomatic nodules or discrete firm, fluctuant swellings within the soft tissues overlying the plantar aspect of one or both feet.

Diagnosis

- Clinical signs and symptoms
- A history of Dupuytren's contracture affecting the hands
- A weak association with alcohol abuse.

Treatment

- None if asymptomatic
- Accommodative orthoses if painful
- Hydrocortisone injections.

Tarsal arthritis

This present with osteoarthritic changes at the midfoot joints with exostoses.

Clinical features

- Pain in the dorsal midfoot
- Palpable thickening of the 1st metatarsal-cuneiform joint
- Loss or reduction of normal movement
- Crepitus
- Overlying tissues may be inflamed
- Dorsal adventitious bursa.

Diagnosis and differential diagnosis

- Plain lateral radiographs of the foot.
  Differential diagnosis includes:
- midtarsal Charcot arthropathy
- midfoot fractures.

Treatment

- Clinical padding
- Footwear advice
- Orthoses
- Surgery.

Plantar fasciitis

This is a common foot problem causing pain in the plantar area of the medial longitudinal arch.

Clinical features

- Pain radiating along the medial band of the plantar fascia
- Pain that is worse on first weight bearing and after periods of prolonged sitting or rest
- Pain that radiates proximally and/or distally within the foot
- Pain induced by standing on tiptoe.

Differential diagnosis

- Heel pain syndrome
- Plantar fibromatosis
- March fracture
- Tibialis posterior dysfunction.

Treatment

- Biomechanical assessment
- Weight loss if required
- Ultrasound therapy
- Anti-pronatory insoles
- A rigid, casted ankle-foot orthosis worn while in bed
- Non-steroidal anti-inflammatory drugs (NSAIDs).

FOREFOOT DISORDERS OR METATARSALGIA

This is a generic term for pain in the metatarsal area.

Pathology and clinical presentation

Abnormal compression forces at the plantar fibro fatty pad of the forefoot are associated with:

- inflexibility of the foot
- fixation of one or more metatarsals or metatarsophalangeal joints
- fixed toe deformity
- subluxation or dislocation of MTPJs.

Treatment

- Identification of the underlying pathomechanical cause of pain
- Gain maximum function of the lesser toes and the MTPJs by:
  - clinical padding
  - correctly fitting shoes
  - functional orthoses
  - surgery.

Non-functional metatarsalgia

This comprises painful forefoot conditions not related to biomechanical problems, e.g. Freiberg's disease and Morton's neuroma.

Metatarsalgia can be considered within broad causative categories:

- relating to soft-tissue pathology:
  - focal plantar hyperkeratosis
  - plantar fibromatosis
  - synovial tissue pathologies, ganglia, adventitious bursae, capsulitis, gouty tophus, rheumatoid bursae and nodules
  - vascular pathologies, ischaemia, venous and lymphatic insufficiency
  - neurological problems, sensory dysfunction, nerve entrapments, neuritis and neuroma
  - muscular pathologies
  - neoplasm
- relating to bone and joint pathology
- relating to systemic pathology.

Focal hyperkeratoses

These are also known as intractable plantar keratoses (IPK), tyloma, heloma vasculare and heloma neurovasculare.

Treatment

For more information see
Neale's Disorders of the Foot 8E   *page 130*

- Ray surgery to correct an associated lesser toe deformity.

Metatarsalgia due to synovial tissue pathology (ganglia/ganglionic cysts)

Due to weakness in the wall of a synovial tendon sheath or a joint capsule.

Pathology

- The tendon sheath or joint capsule herniates.

Clinical picture

- Ganglion shows transillumination
- Swelling has an easily palpable margin
- A 'fluid thrill' within the lesion can be detected.

Treatment

The range of treatments includes:

- direct pressure to the lesion with compression dressings
- application of deflective or cushioning clinical padding
- aspiration of the cystic fluid
- surgical excision of the ganglion
- possible partial joint excision if cyst is formed by herniation of an interphalangeal joint.

Bursae

Adventitious bursae form over bony prominences in relation to local shear stresses. In the long term they may become fibrous, distended, inflamed, infected or even calcified (see Chapter 2).

Capsulitis

This is inflammation of a joint capsule (capsulitis) arising secondarily to oste-oarthritis (OA) and rheumatoid arthritis(RA) or ongoing low grade trauma.

Pathology

The articular synovium associated with joint ligaments and local tendon sheaths become engorged, swollen and softened by the inflammatory process.

Treatment

The condition can be treated by:

- physical therapies
- NSAIDs
- disease-modifying antirheumatic drugs (DMARDs), if RA is present
- resting of the area.

Gouty tophus

Gout is a crystal-deposition disease that predisposes to arthropathy.

Pathology

- Raised levels of uric acid
- Gouty tophi commonly affect distal tissue, e.g. at the 1st MTPJ, the nail bed and the outer margin and pinna of the ear

- The disease tends to affect males over 30 years of age and postmenopausal women.

Clinical picture

- Acute inflammation
- Severe pain in the affected joint
- Pain subsides gradually
- Swelling reduces over time
- Skin of inflamed area may peel off
- Persists as a chronic condition
- Degenerative changes occur within the joint
- Skin overlying tophi may perforate
- Subungual gouty tophi causes onycholysis, subungual breakdown and onychauxis.

Diagnosis

- Blood urate levels and erythrocyte sedimentation rate (ESR) raised
- Radiographs show characteristic 'punched out' erosions at joint margins
- Polarised-light microscopy of aspirated joint fluid shows birefringent crystals.

Treatment

- Drugs to control pain and inflammation (NSAIDs)
- Uricosuric agents to reduce blood urate levels
- Rest or non-weight bearing at the painful area.

Rheumatoid nodules and rheumatoid bursae

Patients with rheumatoid arthritis are prone to develop large adventitious bursae within the plantar tissues overlying the MTPJs and fibrinoid nodules over bony prominences (see Chapter 8).

Plantar plate rupture

Rupture of the tough, rectangular, fibrocartilaginous structure that overlies the plantar aspects of the MTPJs.

Clinical picture

- Increased weight bearing at the forefoot and hyperextension at the MTPJs predisposes to plantar plate dysfunction
- Rupture or attenuation of the plantar plate at the 2nd to 5th MTPJs. More frequent in women, secondary to trauma.
- The condition is associated with:
  - a long second metatarsal
  - a short first metatarsal
  - inflammatory arthropathies
  - diabetes mellitus
  - age-related joint tissues degeneration
  - biomechanical anomalies
  - athletes, who are prone to this condition.

Diagnosis and differential diagnosis

- History and presenting symptoms
- A positive vertical stress test

- Radiograph (arthrography)
- MRI scan.

Differential diagnosis:

- synovitis in association with rheumatological disease
- traumatic subluxation of the toe
- osteochondritis of the metatarsal head
- stress fracture
- plantar digital neuroma.

Treatment

Conservative treatments of plantar plate rupture are designed to:

- ease local pain
- rest the area
- minimise digital deformity.

Conservative measures include:

- taping to maintain correct intra-ray alignment
- clinical plantar pads to dorsiflex the metatarsal and plantarflex the toe
- orthoses to correct any underlying biomechanical faults
- exercises
- NSAIDs
- intra-articular hydrocortisone injection.

Note that pads or orthoses that incorporate a 'U'd' cut out for the affected MTPJ may exacerbate the presenting problem.

Surgery is indicated for cases that fail to respond to conservative therapies. Recommended procedures include:

- osseous correction of the deformed digit
- flexor-to-extensor tendon transfer
- repair of the tear in the plantar plate or collateral ligament.

Neurological problems

Patients with painful neuropathy or hyperalgesia experience:

- radiating, burning, sharp or shooting pains
- symptoms exacerbated by movement
- Tinel's sign
- Valleix' sign
- altered nerve conduction rates
- Note: painful neuropathy or hyperaesthesia may be a feature of diabetic sensory neuropathy.

Nerve entrapment – Morton's neuroma

Morton's neuroma, plantar digital neuroma (PDN), causes spasmodic neurological pain in the forefoot. It is a common condition often affecting middle-aged women.

Neuroma can affect either foot but bilateral presentation is less common. Approximately 90% of cases affect either the $2^{nd}/3^{rd}$ or $3^{rd}/4^{th}$ web spaces and 10% affects the $1^{st}/2^{nd}$ or $4^{th}/5^{th}$ interspaces.

Pathology/aetiology

- Nerve compression and tension especially in the $3^{rd}–4^{th}$ interspace
- Distal extension of the intermetatarsal bursa at toe-off

- Transient nerve ischaemia
- Biomechanical factors.

Clinical picture

- Sudden, sharp, shocking, burning, paroxysmal and spasmodic debilitating pain
- Pain is triggered by prolonged standing, walking or running
- Pain may occur during rest
- Removal of footwear and massage to the foot gives relief
- Pain is aggravated by tight, narrow, thin-soled or high-heeled shoes
- Pain can occur spontaneously and during the night
- Pain radiates into the toes, the dorsum of foot, and/or the lower part of the back of the leg
- Sensation is of walking on a 'lump' or 'pebble'
- Paraesthesia, tingling and numbness of the toes to either side of the affected web space
- Palpable thickening and oedema of the affected webbing area
- Local oedema causes the toes to diverge slightly.

Diagnosis and differential diagnosis

The diagnosis of plantar digital neuroma (PDN) is:

- characteristic presenting symptoms
- pain on lateral compression of the metatarsal heads
- distal parasthesia or hypoaesthesia, e.g. loss of sensation at the affected interdigital space
- temporary reduction of pain by injection of local anaesthetic into the area of the neuroma
- nerve lesion not visible on radiograph, but the lesion is well visualised on MRI and high resolution.

    Nerve conduction tests are inconclusive.
    The differential diagnosis includes:

- forefoot pain arising as the result of: lumbar radiculopathy
- tarsal tunnel syndrome
- metatarsal or stress fracture
- Freiberg's infraction
- peripheral neuritis or neuropathy
- inter-metatarsal bursitis
- arthritides
- metatarsal and soft-tissue tumours
- rupture of the plantar plate
- metatarsophalangeal joint capsulitis.

Treatment

The treatment of plantar digital neuroma should address all aspects of the presenting problem, as well as the associated predisposing factors:

- full biomechanical assessment
- correction of anomalies with clinical anti-pronatory orthoses
- appropriate shoe style
- NSAIDs
- a mix of corticosteroid and local anaesthetic injection
- surgical excision.

Other causes of metatarsalgia

Metatarsalgia may be a presenting feature of a range of other foot and limb pathologies. These include:

- plantar fibromatosis
- intermittent claudication
- rest pain
- impaired venous drainage
- chronic lymphatic insufficiency of the lower limb
- myalgia (fibrositis, fibromyositis, and myositis)
- tendonitis, muscle strains
- neoplastic disease.

Metatarsalgia arising in association with bone pathologies

Stress fractures

Hairline cracks that arise in bone as the result of the repeated application of low-level stresses.

March fracture

Clinical picture

- Symptoms are often mild initially
- Commonly affects the proximal or distal $\frac{1}{3}$ of the 2nd, 3rd or 4th metatarsal shaft
- History of extra exercise or weight increase
- Pain and aching in the metatarsal area after and during exercise
- Local swelling and bruising subside gradually but pain persists
- Wearing high heels exacerbates the symptoms
- Pain when standing on tiptoe.

Diagnosis and differential diagnosis

- History and the appearance of swelling or bruising at the dorsum of the foot
- Fracture not obvious on plain radiograph in early stages
- After 3–4 weeks X-rays show diffuse bone callus at fracture site
- Stress fractures is visible at earliest stage on bone scan.

    The differential diagnosis of a march fracture:

- metatarsal osteochondritis
- bone tumour
- Charcot neuro-arthropathy
- Osteomyelitis.

Treatment

March fractures require immobilisation and protection from weight bearing and ground reaction forces to promote bone healing:

- rest by a below-knee plaster cast or using an Aircast® boot
- immobilisation by soft splints made from clinical padding materials
- the application of elastic tubular bandage, such as Tubigrip®
- clinical strapping
- a shoe with a stiff, curved-profile, or rocker sole.

Other bones in the foot prone to stress fractures:

- calcaneus: a vague heel pain that eludes diagnosis
- sesamoids: stress fractures of the sesamoids may be difficult to differentiate from the presentation of bipartite or enlarged sesamoids
- styloid process of the 5th metatarsal: should be distinguished from Iselin's disease.

Sesamoid pathologies

- Bipartite sesamoids are encountered twice as often as multipartite sesamoids.
- Metatarsalgia at the plantar medial aspect of the 1st MTPJ may may relate to sesamoid pathology.
- Chondromalacia, or dystrophy of articular cartilage is a relatively common cause of sesamoid pathology.
- Sesamoiditis is a common condition that typically affects physically active young girls.

Clinical picture

Signs and symptoms:

- aching
- tenderness
- swelling
- pain increases insidiously, but may develop into a constant throb
- pain on movement, especially dorsiflexion of the great toe at weight-bearing
- soft tissues surrounding the affected sesamoid are tender and inflamed
- pain and swelling limits normal dorsiflexion and plantarflexion at the 1st MTPJ.
- Surgical 'planning' of the affected sesamoid.

Treatment

- Rest with minimal weight bearing
- Deflective clinical padding
- Soft splinting of the first MTPJ
- NSAIDs
- Severe cases require fixed immobilisation in a below-knee walking cast
- Injection of corticosteroid
- Biomechanical assessment to determine the underlying cause.

Sesamoid fractures

Symptoms mimic sesamoiditis such as:

- pain on the plantar aspect of the 1st MTPJ and the medial forefoot area
- swelling
- limited sagittal plane movement of the 1st MTPJ
- patient with a sesamoid fracture presents with a history of traumatic injury.

Following the sesamoid fracture:

- the forefoot becomes very tender, swollen and bruised
- focal pain at the first MTPJ
- fracture is confirmed by plain radiographs
- treated by rest and full immobilisation.

Other causes of metatarsalgia related to bone problems

- Freiberg's infraction
- Complications following metatarsal surgery
- Trauma, surgery, fixation or loss of mobility of joints of 1st ray.

Systemic conditions associated with metatarsalgia

Any generalised pathology that affects the locomotor system is likely to give rise to pain in the foot, and thus can be a cause of metatarsalgia:

- arthropathies
- osteoarthritis
- rheumatoid arthritis
- psoriatic arthritis
- ankylosing spondylitis
- connective tissue disorders
- infective and reactive arthritis
- back pain
- paget's disease
- neoplastic disease
- mucopolysaccharide disorders
- skeletal dysplasia (for example achondroplasia; osteomalacia)
- hereditary diseases such as osteogenesis imperfecta and osteoporosis
- obesity
- later stages of pregnancy
- alcoholism can cause the development of painful neuropathies of the lower limbs and foot.

FIRST RAY PATHOLOGIES

Hallux abducto valgus (HAV)

This is a forefoot pathology which exhibits:

- lateral deviation of the hallux at the 1st MTPJ
- formation of an exostosis and bursa at the medial aspect of the head of the 1st metatarsal
- degenerative changes at 1st MTPJ
- hammer deformity and/or dislocation at 2nd MTPJ
- crowding of the forefoot.

Aetiology

- A strong familial predisposition but is not inherited *per se*
- A range of biomechanical anomalies predisposing to excessive foot pronation.

  The clinical picture of HAV includes:

- fibular deviation of the great toe at the 1st MTPJ
- tibial deviation of the distal part of the 1st metatarsal
- loss or reduction of the normal articular relationships at the 1st MTPJ
- instability of the 1st ray
- structural and soft-tissue pathologies at the 1st MTPJ
- digital crowding and development of lesser toe deformities.

Planar movements at the normal 1st metatarsophalangeal joint

Active movement at the normal 1st MTPJ includes:

- sagittal plane movement (dorsiflexion and plantar flexion)
- transverse plane movement (adduction and abduction)
- no active frontal plane movement (inversion and eversion).

Factors that predispose to the development of hallux abducto valgus

Factors that predispose to the development of HAV include intrinsic features of the lower limb and foot, extrinsic features related to systemic pathology, and certain variants of normal foot anatomy.

Intrinsic factors

- Biomechanical factors leading to excessive pronation at the STJ include:
  - ankle equinus
  - flexible or rigid pes planovalgus
  - rigid or flexible forefoot varus
  - dorsiflexion of the first ray
  - over-long 2nd metatarsal
  - relatively short 1st metatarsal
  - functional hallux limitus
- Structural anomalies within the lower limb that also predispose to compensatory excessive foot pronation and resultant HAV include:
  - external tibial torsion
  - tibial varum
  - positional variants of the knee (genu valgum/varum/recurvatum)
  - femoral retroversion
  - abducted angle of gait or a wide-based gait
  - leg-length discrepancy
- Trauma such as:
  - intra-articular damage within the 1st MTPJ
  - soft-tissue tears and 1st MTPJ sprains
  - dislocation or amputation of the 2nd toe at the 2nd MTPJ.

Extrinsic factors

Extrinsic (systemic) factors associated with an increased incidence of HAV include:

- inflammatory joint disease e.g. RA
- connective tissue disorders and systemic pathologies
- neuromuscular diseases

Variants of normal foot anatomy

There are a number of normal anatomical variants that can exacerbate a tendency towards developing HAV. These include:

- an adductus or atavistic foot
- Long or short 1st metatarsal
- unequal extrinsic muscle function
- idiopathic features.

Clinical features

The patient with HAV may present with any or all of the following:

- pain around the 1st MTPJ
- 1st MTPJ pain exacerbated by activity
- 1st MTPJ pain aggravated by tight or high-heeled shoes
- 1st MTPJ pain relieved by rest or a change of shoe style
- lesser toe deformities e.g. hammered, mallet, clawed, retracted toes
- associated nail pathologies e.g. onychodystrophy, onychauxis, onychogryphosis, onychocryptosis and onychophosis
- difficulty in obtaining shoes to accommodate the increased width of the forefoot
- digital and plantar callosity.

In addition to these symptoms, the following may be seen:

- rearfoot and forefoot varus or valgus
- metatarsus primus varus
- HAV
- medial eminence at the head of the 1st metatarsal often with large medial bursa formation
- reduced range of dorsiflexion at the 1st MTPJ
- pain and/or crepitus at the 1st MTPJ on passive movement of the hallux.

Clinical examination

- Ascertain aetiology, where possible
- Biomechanical evaluation of foot and lower limb
  - Hip, knee and ankle alignment
  - Femoral and tibial alignment
  - Ankle joint range of motion
  - ranges of motion at the subtalar and midtarsal joints
  - neutral relaxed calcaneal stance position
  - relationship of the calcaneus to the lower leg at STJ neutral
  - relationship of the forefoot and rearfoot at STJ neutral
  - ranges of motion of the 1st ray and the 1st MTPJ
  - metatarsal formula.

Non-weight-bearing examination

The following should be assessed:

- position of the hallux in relation to the 2nd toe
- Medial eminence at 1st MTPJ
- available range of motion at the 1st MTPJ
- range of motion at the 1st ray
- prominence and course of extensor hallucis longus tendon
- presence of plantar keratoses
- presence of digital keratoses
- presence of paraesthesia or reduced sensation at the medial and dorsomedial quadrant of the hallux
- presence of pain/onychophosis and/or onychocryptosis, at the hallux nail
- presence of other forefoot deformities that form the classic clinical presentation of HAV.

Standing examination

All features of HAV deformity are increased on weight-bearing and exaggerated when the patient stands on tiptoes. In particular the following should be noted:

- hallux abduction and hallux eversion
- angulation of the 1st metatarsal
- contracture of the extensor digitorum longus tendon
- hallux purchase.

Diagnosis of hallux abducto valgus

The diagnosis of HAV is based on:

- clinical observation of the typical deformities e.g. 1st ray misalignments, lesser toe deformities
- hyperkeratotic skin lesions
- reported pain in and around the 1st MTPJ
- metatarsalgia
- the differential diagnoses should exclude inflammatory joint disease and other extrinsic factors that predispose to HAV.

Management of HAV

Management of nail and soft-tissue pathologies

- Reduction of onychauxic nails and sharp debridement
- Regular sharp debridement of corn and hyperkeratosis
- The use of deflective and cushioning digital padding (see Chapter 16)
- Appropriate shoe style (see Chapter 18)
- The provision of bespoke or semi-bespoke shoes if required (see Chapter 18)
- Footwear adaptations (see Chapter 18)
- Orthotic therapy and palliative and dynamic orthoses (see Chapter 17).

Surgical correction of the forefoot deformity

Surgery for HAV:

- soft-tissue surgery
- 1st MTPJ-preserving surgery
- 1st MTPJ-destructive surgery.

Hallux limitus/rigidus

This is a progressive pathology characterised by restriction of dorsiflexion of the hallux and degenerative changes to the 1st MTPJ.

Hallux limitus (HL) may be structural and/or functional.

- Structural hallux limitus: limitation at the 1st MTPJ at all times
- Functional hallux limitus: dorsiflexion at the 1st MTPJ is only reduced during weight-bearing

Aetiology

Intrinsic factors

- Foot shape. The rectus foot is more prone to develop hallux limitus
- Biomechanical factors. These include:
  - ankle equinus
  - flexible or rigid pes planovalgus
  - rigid or flexible forefoot varus
  - dorsiflexion of the 1st ray
  - elevated or hypermobile 1st ray
  - flexor plate immobility
  - plantar soft tissue contracture
  - functional hallux limitus

- Limb and foot anomalies. These include:
  - external tibial torsion
  - tibial varum
  - positional variants of the knee
  - femoral retroversion
  - leg-length discrepancy
  - an abducted angle of gait or wide-based gait
  - A relatively long first toe or long 1st metatarsal
  - Trauma, damage to the articular cartilage at the 1st MTPJ
  - Soft-tissue tears and sprains.

Extrinsic (systemic) factors

- Inflammatory joint disease within the foot
- Occupations requiring repeated and constant forced dorsiflexion of the hallux
- Short shoes.

Pain associated with hallux limitus (HL) and hallux rigidus (HR)

The presenting symptoms of hallux limitus and hallux rigidus vary depending on the stage of the pathology:

Stage 1 – The 1st MTPJ is often asymptomatic

Stage 2 – Patients usually complain of pain in and around the 1st MTPJ under load e.g. on walking

Stage 3 – The 1st MTPJ is painful most of the time

Stage 4 – There is minimal or no movement at the 1st MTPJ due to osteophytosis and the loss of normal bony architecture at the joint, all movement is painful. The 1st MTPJ becomes pain-free when ankylosis is complete.

Shoe wear marks

Characteristic wear marks may be seen in the upper and on the sole of the shoe, more readily seen in a lace up shoe with leather upper and sole (see chapter 18). Shoes show:

Stage 1 – Signs of excessive foot pronation

Stage 2 – Bulging in the upper overlying osteophytosis at the 1st MTPJ. 'Spin' wear on the sole

Stage 3 – Lateral wears on the sole, wear beneath the 1st and 2nd MTPJs, a diagonal crease on the upper

Stage 4 – Marked wear along the medial area of the sole, medial 'bulging' of the upper in the area of the throat of the shoe. Horizontal creases near the top line of the outer side of the lateral area of the heel counter and scratch marks on the outer medial side of the heel.

Diagnosis and differential diagnosis

The diagnosis of hallux limitus and hallux rigidus is made from:

- clinical signs and symptoms
- radiographs.

  Differential diagnosis should rule out inflammatory joint diseases including:

- rheumatoid arthritis
- gout

- psoriatic arthropathy
- osteochondritis dissecans
- flexor hallucis longus tenosynovitis.

Treatment

Hallux limitus and hallux rigidus can be treated conservatively or by surgery. Conservative treatments include:

- clinical reduction of hyperkeratoses e.g. below 2nd, $4^{th}/5^{th}$ MTPJs
- manipulation of affected joint
- manipulation
- shoe-style adaptations
- orthoses for cases of functional hallux limitus to control the abnormal pronatory forces
- functional orthoses for cases with structural hallux limitus, which include accommodation for the 1st metatarsal head.

Indicative staged conservative treatments include the following:

Stage 1 – Functional hallux limitus:
- essentially prophylactic treatment
- orthoses to stabilise the hypermobile 1st ray
- manipulation to maintain the normal range of motion at the 1st MTPJ.

Stage 2 – Mild structural hallux limitus:
- range of motion (ROM) of the 1st MTPJ may be reduced by up to 50%
- if X-ray is normal at *stage 2*, structural hallux limitus is treated as *stage 1* presentation
- degenerative changes at 1st MTPJ – NSAIDs advised
- prescription orthoses to stabilise rear foot and midfoot function.

Stage 3 – Moderate structural hallux limitus:
- ROM of 1st MTPJ reduced by up to 75% – conservative treatment includes
- conservative treatment
- manipulative therapy carried out daily, preceded by the application of heat and followed by the application of an ice pack
- fan strapping to the joint (see Chapter 16)
- ultrasound therapy or iontophoresis
- A painful joint should be:
  - rested by a rocker soled shoe
  - immobilised by the use of Low Dye® strapping
- NSAIDs as necessary
- antipronatory in-shoe orthoses.

Stage 4 – Severe structural hallux limitus/rigidus:
- immobilised with an orthosis
- use of a rocker-soled shoe to allow relatively normal gait in a foot with little or no 1st MTPJ movement.

Surgical treatment of hallux limitus and hallux rigidus

Corrective surgery for structural hallux limitus is recommended when conservative therapies have failed to reduce pain and improve foot function. Surgery includes:

- cheilectomy with the reduction of pressure within the joint by shortening the 1st metatarsal
- arthroplasty and/or the insertion of a 1st MTPJ prosthetic joint replacement
- plantar basal closing wedge osteotomy to realign the first metatarsal
- arthrodesis of the 1st MTPJ.

Hallux flexus

This was formerly referred to as acute hallux rigidus/limitus. An acute presentation of hallux limitus can occur, usually in a younger person as the result of sudden local trauma to the 1st MTPJ. With appropriate treatment, the acute hallux limitus or hallux flexus condition will resolve completely.

Pathology

- Recent history of trauma to the foot
- Acute local pain and inflammatory response I and around the joint
- Flexor hallucis brevis muscle goes into spasm creating a metatarsus primus elevatus
- Hallux remains in plantarflexion until the pain, inflammation and muscle spasm subside
- Repeated episodes of hallux flexus predispose to structural hallux limitus in later life.

Diagnosis

- Clinical signs and symptoms
- Patient history
- Radiographs exclude any fractures caused at the time of the original trauma.

Treatment

Treatment involves RICE:

Rest
- Non weight-bearing regime
- Joint immobilisation achieved by:
  - a shoe with a stiff/non-bending or rocker
  - strapping the 1st MTPJ
  - soft splinting of the 1st MTPJ and forefoot to restrict 1st MTPJ movement.

Ice
- Used in the first 48–72 hours following injury:
  - applied to the inflamed area at least twice a day (see Chapter 16)
  - after 72 hours the application of gentle heat is indicated by immersion in a water bath at 45°C for 10 minutes twice daily use of an infrared lamp a hot-water bottle.

Compression
- Compression bandaging, such as Coban or crepe bandage:
  - applied as a 'figure-of-eight' foot bandage from above the ankle to distal to the MTPJs (see Chapter 16).

Elevation
- Limb fully supported along its length, heel higher than the buttocks.

Pain control must be considered along with RICE treatment e.g. by the prescription of NSAIDs.

Chapter | 5 |

Circulatory disorders

Circulatory disorders of the lower limb can be broadly classified as arterial (macrovascular) or capillary (microvascular) disease, which results in ischaemia, or by venous or lymphatic disease, which impairs venous drainage of blood and interstitial fluid. Fig 5.1

ARTERIOSCLEROSIS (HARDENING OF THE ARTERIES)

Definition: age-related changes in which intima and media of arterial wall becomes thickened and fibrosed, replacement of smooth muscle and elastic fibres of the media with collagen.

Effect: increased rigidity and tortuosity of vessel, contributing to age-related increase in blood pressure.

ATHEROSCLEROSIS (MACROVASCULAR DISEASE)

Definition: thickening of intima of large- and medium-sized arteries, consequent narrowing of artery because of lipid and fibrous deposition.

Effect: progressive narrowing/occlusion of the arteries resulting in ischaemia of tissues supplied by that diseased vessel: atheromas serve as sites for thrombus formation which can result in acute symptoms.

Pathology and epidemiology.

For more information see
Neale's Disorders of the Foot 8E *page 146*

Risk factors: Fig 5.2

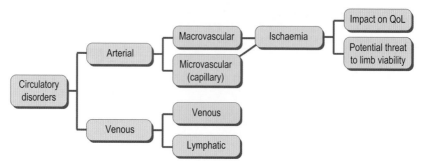

Figure 5.1 Disorders of circulation.

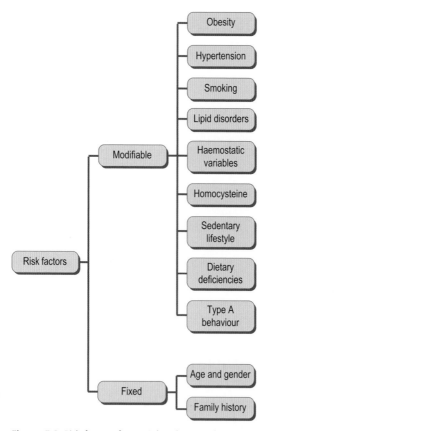

Figure 5.2 Risk factors for peripheral artery disease.

Clinical features

The three cardinal features of symptomatic peripheral arterial disease are:

- intermittent claudication (pain on walking, relieved by rest: usually calfs, but can be buttocks, sole of foot), symptoms being cramping, tightness and loss of power
- rest pain (usually at night, excruciating and burning – relieved by dependent position, not walking)

- gangrene, each of which reflects an increasing degree of ischaemia:
  - cold feet
  - colour changes – pallor, cyanosis.

Physical signs

- Decreased or absent peripheral pulses below the site of obstruction
- Premature limb blanching when the limb is elevated from the supine position
- Ruddy cyanotic hue which spreads over the lower limbs within 3 minutes when the limb is placed in a dependent position from elevation
- Increased capillary filling time (>10 seconds).

Additional physical signs might include: nail changes, e.g. thickening, slow nail plate growth through to loss of the nail plate with scarring; atrophic skin changes characterised by anhidrosis; and thinning of skin and loss of subcutaneous tissues.

Critical limb ischaemia

This describes an advanced stage of peripheral artery disease (PAD), which is regarded as limb-threatening ischaemia.

Diagnosis

Diagnosis of PAD in primary care is frequently based on the clinical method which includes:

- medical
- examination of peripheral pulses
- presenting symptoms – intermittent claudication/rest pain
- presenting signs – cold limb with lack of hair, translucent atrophic skin with or without ulceration, infection and gangrene
- ankle-brachial index
- segmental systolic pressure
- Doppler sounds/spectral wave analysis
- venous filling time
- Buerger's test
- capillary refill time.

> **For more information see**
> Neale's Disorders of the Foot 8E   *pages 148–152*

Specialist vascular laboratory investigations may include:

- digital subtraction arteriography
- duplex ultrasound
- magnetic resonance angiography
- CT angiography
- treadmill exercise testing
- assessment of skin blood.

Visual indications of disease include:

- pink and warm – adequate flow and oxygen saturation
- red and warm – high flow and oxygenation, for example seen in inflammation or abnormal shunting
- cyanotic and cold – decrease in flow and oxygen saturation

- red and cold – reduced perfusion
- white – occlusion either fixed or vasospasm
- black – tissue necrosis.

Classification of peripheral artery disease

Based on symptoms, e.g. claudication distance, ankle–brachial index, critical limb ischaemia (CLI) criteria or the Fontaine classification. The Fontaine classification consists of four stages:

Stage I – Asymptomatic
Stage II – Intermittent claudication
Stage III – Rest pain/nocturnal pain
Stage IV – Necrosis/gangrene.

Clinical management

The focus of management must be on reducing cardiovascular complications, managing pain and improving quality of life (see Figure 5.2 for risk factors that can be reduced).

VASCULITIS

This comprises a group of mixed conditions which are characterised by local inflammation of the walls of arteries or arterioles, with the inflammation extending to affect veins and capillaries in some cases:

- thromboangiitis obliterans
- polyarteritis nodosa
- vasculitis seen in association with rheumatoid arthritis.

Thromboangiitis obliterans (Beurger's disease)

- A perivascular inflammation involving distal arteries, veins and nerves frequently agglutinated by fibrous tissue.

Epidemiology

- The typical age at onset is between 20 and 45 years of age, with males being affected 7–8 times more than females.

Aetiology

- Exact aetiology remains unknown; it is now considered to be an accelerated form of atheroma which affects heavy-smoking young males. There is a slight genetic predisposition associated with HLA A9 & B5.

Clinical features

These include superficial migratory thrombophlebitis, cool dysaesthetic feet, claudication or rest pain, and gangrene. Arterial disease presents in both lower and upper limbs. Features typically include cold feet/hands, paraesthesia, claudication, severe rest pain, and trophic ulceration and gangrene. Claudication, if present, is typically located to intrinsic foot muscles and this symptom is often misdiagnosed as metatarsalgia of orthopaedic origin. Proximal limb pulses are usually normal with distal ones being absent or diminished.

Differential diagnosis

The differential diagnosis is from premature atherosclerosis. Features which assist in differentiating thromboangiitis obliterans from premature atherosclerosis include:

- early onset of symptoms (before 45 years)
- evidence of addictive smoking
- inflammation
- evidence of distal diseases
- involvement of vein and associated nerve
- upper-limb ischaemia
- exclusion of other risk factors.

Treatment

- Stopping smoking arrests development of the disease
- Adequate pain relief
- Acute cases may require hospitalisation for anticoagulant therapy and/or amputation
- Good management of trophic ulcerations
- Careful attention to foot hygiene.

Prognosis

Prognosis is poorer for the foot than the hand.

Polyarteritis nodosa

Polyarteritis nodosa (PAN) is a necrotising vasculitis affecting medium-sized arteries. It affects twice as many males as females and peak incidence is in the fourth and fifth decades of life.

Clinical features

Classical signs include vague systemic illness, muscle pains, mononeuritis multiplex, abdominal pains, severe hypertension, chest pain, renal impairment, arthritis, claudication and cutaneous lesions such as palpable purpura, ulceration and gangrene.

Differential diagnosis

This is mainly from other collagen vascular disorders that can produce indistinguishable lesions. The diagnosis is based on clinical features; angiography shows multiple aneurysms and smooth narrowing of affected vessels.

Treatment

Antiviral therapy or immunosuppressive therapy is beneficial in most cases.

Rheumatoid vasculitis

Vasculitis is seen in approximately 20% of patients with rheumatoid arthritis who present with nodules and are positive for rheumatoid factor. Vasculitis affects small vessels resulting in nail fold infarcts and small areas of tissue ulceration; small arteries, responsible for larger areas of cutaneous ulceration and digital gangrene. In some patients the usual signs of vaculitis (skin infarction, neuropathy and scleritis) may be absent.

The key features may be rapid weight loss, fever, malaise and persistently raised erythrocyte sedimentation rate (ESR).

VASOSPASTIC DISORDERS

Raynaud's phenomenon

Raynaud's phenomenon describes any form of cold-related vasospasm and can be subdivided into:

- raynaud's disease (RD) – when the symptoms are consistent with the original description and where connective tissue disease is absent both clinically and serologically
- raynaud's syndrome (RS) – where there is an associated disease.

Raynaud's disease is a common condition occurring in 5–10% of the population and it is especially common in women aged 20–40 years of age. The range of disorders associated with Raynaud's syndrome is wide and includes the following.

Immune mediated

- Systemic sclerosis (affects 95% of patients)
- Systemic lupus erythematosus (affects 10–45% of patients)
- Mixed connective tissue disease (affects 85% of patients)
- Polymyositis/dermatomyositis (affects 20% of patients)
- Sjögren's syndrome (affects 33% of patients)
- Rheumatoid arthritis (affects 10% of patients)
- Cryoglobulinaemias.

Drug induced

- Anti-migraine compounds
- Cytotoxic drugs
- Beta blockers (particularly non-selective).

Occupation related

- Vibration exposure (affects up to 50% of workers)
- Cold injury (frozen food packers)
- Polyvinyl chloride exposure.

Obstructive vascular disease

- Atherosclerosis
- Micro-emboli
- Thromboangiitis obliterans
- Thoracic outlet syndrome.

Clinical features

On exposure to cold/change in temperature, typically two or three fingers or toes (in up to 50% of cases) go into a prolonged vasospasm, initially turn white and then feel numb with a progressive loss of fine movement. This is followed by cyanosis, which is due to a slow blood flow and desaturation, and, finally, the affected fingers or toes turn bright red and painful from a reactive hyperaemia.

Treatment

- Prevention and self-management, e.g. avoiding cold exposure and using heated gloves
- Vasodilator therapy, e.g. nifedipine
- In severe cases prostaglandin analogues.

For other rare conditions which might affect the feet and legs refer to the main text, e.g. acrocyanosis, erythomelalgia, livedo reticularis, erythema abigne, frost-bite and immersion foot (trench foot).

MICROVASCULAR DISEASE

Microvascular disease occurs in both insulin-dependent and non-insulin-dependent diabetes mellitus, and its development is linked to the duration of diabetes and the degree of glycaemic control. The term microvascular disease refers to the changes seen in the smallest vessels, capillaries and arterioles. The resultant effect is decreased blood flow and reduced vasodilatory capacity.

Wound healing is impaired and the tissue's ability to respond to traumatic incidents and invasion of micro-organisms is limited.

Venous disease

This comprises thrombosis and thrombophilia (inherited or acquired state leading to increased risk of thromoembolic disease).

Thrombosis (homeostasis in the wrong place) requires two of the following three states (Virchow's triad):

- blood stasis:
  - all conditions with immobility
  - impaired limb mobility
  - congestive heart failure
  - compression of a vein, e.g. pressure from a tumour or abscess
- alteration to the vein wall:
  - history of previous thrombosis
  - inflammation/infection around the vein
  - direct vein wall trauma, e.g. cannula or surgical trauma
  - varicose veins
- hypercoagulability states:
  - deficiencies in, e.g., antithrombin, protein S and protein C
  - antiphospholipid syndrome
  - hyperhomocysteinaemia
  - surgery (especially lower-limb surgery), trauma and injury
  - childbirth
  - polycythaemia
  - neoplastic disease
  - oral contraceptive (oestrogen therapy).

The clinical presentation of venous thromboembolic disease varies:

- deep venous thrombosis (DVT), typically affecting the calf veins
- pulmonary embolism as a secondary complication of DVT
- recurrent DVT
- atypical thrombosis in the cerebral, axillary and mesenteric veins
- recurrent mid-trimester fetal loss.

Deep venous thrombosis (DVT)

This is a common and important condition which should be recognised early in its development and have diagnosis confirmed. Failure to diagnose and instigate effective treatment may result in pulmonary embolism which could be fatal, and permanent damage and impairment of lower-limb venous drainage.

The profile of the patient is likely to include increasing age, obesity, pregnancy, history of previous thrombosis and/or surgery (frequently hip and knee surgery), and use of oral contraceptives.

Clinical diagnosis

Diagnosis is notoriously difficult and is prone to false positives. Objective tests include diagnostic imaging (venography, ultrasound, plethysmography, spiral CT or MRI) and haematological assays.

Clinical features

A common site is the calf: in the posterior tibial and peroneal veins, and then in the femoral vein and the iliofemoral vein, which produce the most severe manifestations because of the proximal position.

Other clinical features include the following:

- silent in up to 50% of cases
- often starts 3–10 days post surgery
- involves slight pyrexia
- mild pain in the calf made worse by exercise
- swelling distal to the thrombosis
- distension of the superficial veins
- slight increase in tissue temperature distal to the clot
- cyanotic colour to the distal tissues
- positive Homan's sign (pain in the calf on ankle dorsiflexion)
- symptoms of pulmonary embolism.

Differential diagnosis

- Muscle injury
- Baker's cyst (compressing the popliteal vein)
- Contusion of the calf muscle
- Cellulitis
- Arthritis
- Oedema due to other causes.

Treatment

Aims of treatment are to prevent: propagation of the thrombosis, pulmonary embolism and valvular damage, which could lead to long-term impairment of venous drainage. Treatment will include:

- physical measures:
  - bed rest (limb elevated) for 1 week, as this is the time taken to stabilise the clot
  - elastic stocking to reduce swelling and protect the superficial veins
  - 3–6 months, limitation of prolonged standing.
- anticoagulants – Mainstay of treatment which prevents thrombus extension, new thrombus formation and embolisation of the thrombosis and reduces the complications of developing pulmonary embolism:
  - heparin – administered either subcutaneously or intravenously for 6–8 days depending on the extent of the thrombosis. Should be continued

until the international normalised ratio (INR) is >2.0 for 2 consecutive days.
  - warfarin therapy will commence at the same time as it takes 2–3 days to decrease the concentration of the vitamin K-dependent clotting factors.
- thrombolysis:
  - thrombolytic agents – designed to dissolve the thrombus and should only be considered with significant proximal thrombosis where DVT is considered a significant risk.
- surgical:
  - vena caval filters – mechanical devices which prevent emboli reaching the lungs.

Pulmonary thromboembolism

The most common origin of a pulmonary embolism is a DVT in the legs (80%) followed by thrombosis in the pelvis (15%).

Features of pulmonary thromboembolism include the following:

- small embolus:
  - dyspnoea on excursion
  - tiredness
  - cardiac arrhythmias (rare)
- medium-size embolus:
  - pleuritic pain
  - cough and haemoptysis
  - dyspnoea
- massive embolus:
  - chest pain
  - shock
  - tachycardia
  - acute right-sided cardiac failure
  - death.

Superficial thrombophlebitis

This is a common/recurring problem seen in primary care that presents with a local area of skin around a superficial vein being tender, swollen, warm and red. The vein feels indurated and resistant to light finger compression. Onset is often sudden and triggered by direct trauma to the vein.

Treatment

It does not require anticoagulation. Analgesics and non-steroidal anti-inflammatory drugs (NSAIDs) combined with correct compression therapy (compression is contraindicated in a patient with PAD with an ankle brachial pressure index (ABPI) value of <0.8) and an exercise walking regimen. Antibiotics should only be used when there is evidence of infection.

Chronic venous stasis

This is a common condition and results from either extensive or repeated venous thrombosis and/or valvular incompetence associated with varicose veins or a failure in the venous pump mechanism/s.

Clinical features

- Pain on standing (often described as a bursting sensation which is relived with elevation)
- Oedema (initially pitting but becoming non-pitting with chronicity)
- Cyanotic appearance
- Lipodermatosclerosis (due to the leakage of fibrinogen through the vessel wall which gets converted into the fibrin cuff, which tightens the skin and gives the leg the shape of an inverted bottle of champagne)
- Reduced ankle movement (due to the fibrin cuff)
- Atrophie blanche (white irregular-shaped areas of tissue with one or two dilated capillaries visible, this is slow necrosis of tissue and the potential site of venous ulceration)
- Telangiectasia (dilated capillaries)
- Ulceration (typically located to the lower third of the leg on the medial and lateral sides)
- Lichenification (excessive scales often due to continual bandaging which interferes with desquamation)
- Dermatitis (frequently caused by topical medication).

Treatment

Treatment directed at reducing venous hypertension by compression therapy and regular exercise walking regimens, and, where possible, limb elevation to aid venous drainage. Surgical ligation, stripping and local sclerosing agents may be a long-term cure.

LYMPHATIC DISEASE

Lymphoedema

Primary lymphoedema (Milroy's disease)

This is caused by a failure in the development or an absence of lymphatic vessels in embryonic life. It is seen in isolation or in association with other congenital anomalies, e.g. Turner's syndrome. The development of the oedema is insidious and the age at onset will reflect the varying degrees of failure. Lymphograms show varying degrees of hypoplasia or even aplasia in the main vessels or, less frequently, there may be gross varicose dilatations and reflux into the skin.

There are three different subtypes:

- congenital lymphoedema – appears at or near birth
- lymphoedema praecox – appears after birth and before 35 years of age (typically at puberty)
- lymphoedema tarda – lymphoedema after the age of 35 years.

Secondary lymphoedema

Secondary lymphoedema is due to an obstruction of the lymphatic vessels by some known pathological process:

- filariasis – parasitic worms indigenous to West Africa, India, and part of South America, cause an allergic lymphangitis. Recurrent episodes may lead to lymphatic obstruction and lymphoedema which may affect the legs, arms, breast and genitalia, and may become permanent. This condition is also known as elephantiasis

- malignant disease – due to infiltration of the vessels and nodes by tumour cells or by compression of the vessels
- radiotherapy – causes obstruction and fibrosis of the vessels
- trauma
- chronic infection.

Clinical features

The age of onset varies and in secondary lymphoedema it depends upon the underlying cause. Primary lymphoedema affects both sexes, though the majority is female. Cases usually present before 35 years with features developing in one lower limb. Initially it is the pitting type, which is reduced with elevation, but eventually it becomes non-pitting and indurated as a result of fibrosis. The epidermis is classically 'warty and hyperkeratotic in appearance'.

Diagnosis

This is based on clinical history and presentation, and on the exclusion of other cause(s) of oedema. Lymphangiograms are a definitive test to confirm lymphatic obstruction.

Treatment

- Eliminating the underlying cause where possible, e.g. treatment of chronic infections
- Encourage limb elevation, compression therapy and exercise
- Pneumatic massaging devices, e.g. Flowtron boots
- Careful attention to skin hygiene
- Diuretic therapy
- Microsurgical techniques to improve drainage (these are continuing to be developed).

Chapter | 6 |

Neurological disorders in the lower extremity

THE SPINAL CORD PATHWAYS AND CLINICAL EXAMINATION

Ascending pathways

- Using a biothesiometer, a patient who does not feel vibration at a setting of 25 is considered to be at risk for neurotrophic injury. Fig 6.1
- Decreased vibratory sense is associated with several disease processes, most notably diabetes mellitus, alcohol abuse, vitamin B_{12} deficiencies and tabes dorsalis.
- Vibratory sense decreases with the normal ageing process and patients over the age of 50 may have a measurable level of decrease in sensation distally. Care should be taken to separate this loss from that of true dorsal column pathology.
- Proprioception can be assessed by asking the patient, with eyes closed, to determine whether the hallux is dorsiflexed or plantarflexed.
- Light touch can be evaluated by passing a wisp of cotton over the dermatomes of the foot. The patient should not be 'tickled' as this represents evaluation of subliminal pain.
- Evaluation of pain sensation is performed by pricking the patient over the various dermatomes of the extremity with a moderately sharp needle. Any area of decreased sensation should be carefully mapped out and compared from distal to proximal and bilaterally.
- Temperature may be evaluated with an alcohol-saturated swab. The swab is squeezed to trickle a small amount over the foot. The patient is then asked to identify the cold sensation associated with the evaporation of the alcohol.
- To test for a cerebellar lesion the heel-to-shin test is the most reliable clinical indicator. Place the patient in a supine position and ask to place the heel of one foot on the contralateral knee or shin and draw the heel distally along the shin which should display smooth and even movement. Awkwardness or an inability to place the heel on the knee is suggestive of cerebellar disease.

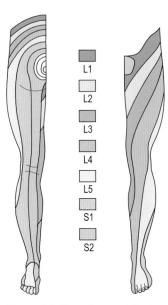

Figure 6.1 Dermatomes of the lower extremity.

- Romberg's test may be used asking the patient to stand with feet close together and with eyes closed. In the presence of cerebellar pathology the patient will sway.

Descending pathways

- Evaluation of the voluntary motor system includes muscle power, bulk and tone with note taken of any involuntary movements such as fasciculations or tremors, chorea or athetosis.
- Movement is assessed for smoothness and co-ordination. Deep tendon reflex responses are evaluated. Fig 6.2
- A Babinski sign is virtually pathognomonic for the presence of an upper motor neuron lesion when present beyond the age of 2 years.
- Clonus is associated with increased muscle tone and hyper-reflexia and reflects the presence of a corticospinal tract lesion. Ankle joint clonus is elicited by a quick, vigorous dorsiflexion of the foot with the knee held in flexion. Greater than three beats suggests nerve injury. Table 6.1

Peripheral entrapment neuropathies

- Proximal tarsal tunnel syndrome is a result of entrapment of the posterior tibial nerve or its branches occurring under the flexor retinaculum. Fig 6.3
- Clinical presentation, regardless of the underlying aetiology, is a symptom complex of tingling, burning and numbness along the plantar aspect of the foot.
- These symptoms may be reproduced with percussion of the posterior tibial nerve at the level of the flexor retinaculum.
- The patient usually has a flexible flat foot with concomitant gastrocnemius-soleus equinus.
- Distal tarsal tunnel syndrome reflects the entrapment of the medial or lateral plantar nerves and may be referred to as 'jogger's foot'.

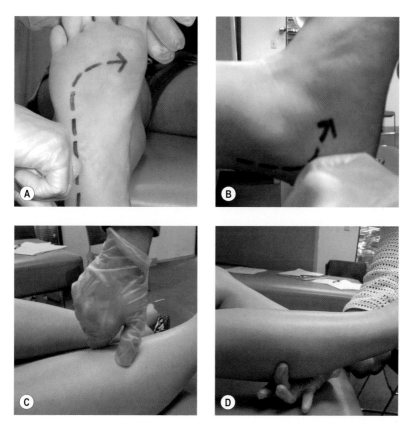

Figure 6.2 Pathological reflex responses. Technique for eliciting the Babinski response (A). Alternative methods include: (B) the Chaddock reflex response elicited by stroking behind the fibular malleolus from proximal to distal; (C) the Oppenheim reflex response elicited by stroking the tibial crest using the fingers as calipers from proximal to distal; and (D) the Gordon reflex response, elicited by squeezing the posterior calf. All of the reflex responses, when present, will demonstrate flexing and fanning of the lesser digits.

Table 6.1 Percussion responses		
TENDON PERCUSSED	**SPINAL NERVE ROOTS**	**REFLEX RESPONSE**
Biceps brachialis	C5–C6	Flexion of forearm
Triceps brachialis	C7–C8	Extension of forearm
Patellar	L3–L4	Knee joint extension
Achilles	S1–S2	Ankle joint plantarflexion

- Irritation of a *plantar intermetatarsal nerve* may lead to the development of a neuroma; an enlargement of the nerve at the level of the metatarsal heads.
- Symptoms may be described as tingling, burning or numbness and radiate distally into the digits. High-heeled or tight-fitting shoe gear exacerbates the discomfort.

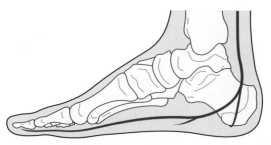

Figure 6.3 Branches of the posterior tibial nerve. The medial calcaneal, medial plantar and lateral plantar branches of the posterior tibial nerve are illustrated.

Table 6.2 Results of nerve trunk irritation in the foot	
INVOLVED NERVE	**NOMENCLATURE**
Medial plantar digital proper	Joplin's neuroma
1st plantar intermetatarsal nerve	Houser's neuroma
2nd plantar intermetatarsal nerve	Heuter's neuroma
3rd plantar intermetatarsal nerve	Morton's neuroma
4th plantar intermetatarsal nerve	Islen's neuroma

- Clinically, direct palpation of the nerve or compression of the metatarsals (Mulder's sign) will reproduce the patient's symptoms; the digits innervated by the intermetatarsal nerve may appear separated from each other (Sullivan's sign).
- Any of the plantar intermetatarsal nerves may be involved, but the third is most common. Table 6.2
- The common peroneal nerve is very vulnerable to compression injuries. Fig 6.4
- Neuropraxia can occur simply from crossing one's legs.
- Iatrogenic injury may occur secondary to positioning on the operating room table or the placement of a below-the-knee cast where the proximal edge impinges on the nerve with knee joint flexion.
- Blunt trauma to the area or traction on the nerve from an inversion ankle injury can cause pathology.
- Clinical findings include muscular weakness of the lateral and anterior compartments creating a drop foot deformity.
- The superficial peroneal nerve may become entrapped. Fig 6.5
- Symptoms may be reproduced with dorsiflexion and eversion of the ankle joint against resistance and direct percussion of the nerve where it exits the fascia.
- The intermediate dorsal cutaneous nerve is extremely susceptible to damage with inversion ankle injuries and with ankle arthroscopy.
- The medial dorsal cutaneous nerve may be compressed by shoes, often at the level of the first metatarsal cuneiform joint.
- The deep peroneal nerve (anterior tibial nerve), becomes damaged between the extensor hallucis longus and extensor digitorum longus tendons and is known as anterior tarsal syndrome.

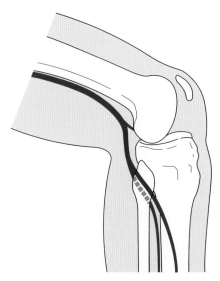

Figure 6.4 Common peroneal nerve at the level of the head and neck of the fibula.

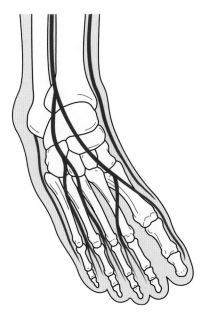

Figure 6.5 Bifurcation of the superficial peroneal nerve into the medial and intermediate dorsal cutaneous nerves.

- Aetiological factors include exostoses of the tarsal bones and tight or ill-fitting shoes, particularly ski boots and high-topped shoes, which demonstrate a maximum point of contact at the dorsal talonavicular joint.
- Patients will present with a complaint of paraesthesias over the dorsal aspect of the foot and numbness within the first intermetatarsal space.
- Injury of the sural nerve occurs at the level of the ankle joint, iatrogenically with a surgeon's 'slip of the hand' or from fibrosis secondary to an inversion ankle injury.

Hereditary motor and sensory neuropathies

- Charcot–Marie–Tooth disease type I is also referred to as peroneal muscular atrophy. It is an autosomal dominantly inherited disorder which results from a mutation in the gene coding for peripheral myelin protein-22 on chromosome 17:
  - onset usually between the ages of 5 and 15 years
  - difficulty in walking, muscle cramps and paraesthesias in the legs
  - development of a high-arched or cavus-appearing foot
  - clawed toe deformities develop. Fig 6.6
  - flaccid paralysis develops, frequently with fascicular twitching in the wasting muscles

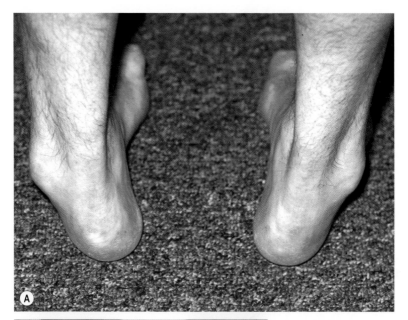

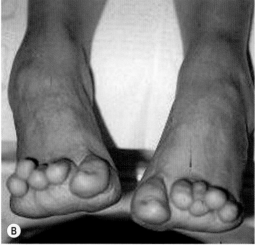

Figure 6.6 Charcot–Marie–Tooth disease. (A) View from rear. (B) View from front.

- Deep tendon reflex responses are decreased or completely absent
- Lower extremities are observed as slender legs with plump thighs and are often described as 'an inverted champagne bottle' or 'ostrich legs'
- roussy–Levy syndrome is also known as hereditary areflexic dystasia:
  - transmitted as an autosomal dominant trait
  - symptoms generally develop in early childhood
  - characterised by the presence of an essential tremor
  - similar clinically to Charcot–Marie–Tooth disease
  - sensory ataxia or poor judgement of movement
  - distal muscular atrophy of the peroneal muscles and a kyphoscoliosis
- dejerine–Sottas disease is also known as Charcot–Marie–Tooth disease type III or as hypertrophic polyneuritis:
  - autosomal recessive inheritance with onset of symptoms occurring in early infancy
  - more severe than type I
  - delayed motor milestones, poor walking and an inability to run
  - distal muscular weakness with peroneal atrophy resulting in a cavus foot deformity
- refsum's disease is also known as Charcot–Marie–Tooth disease type IV:
  - extremely rare autosomal recessive disorder
  - presents as a triad of retinitis pigmentosa, peripheral neuropathy and cerebellar ataxia
  - onset generally occurs within the first years of life
  - lower extremity manifestations of progressive distal neuropathy leading to cavus foot deformity, foot drop and cerebellar ataxia.

Spinal radiculopathies

- Radiculopathy – pathology pertaining to the spinal nerve roots and is secondary to irritation, inflammation or trauma involving the fifth lumbar or first sacral nerve distribution.
- Radicular pain may present as focal irritation of a nerve root or 'local', visceral pain secondary to nerve root irritation, or 'referred' pain, which follows the distribution of the nerve involved or 'radicular'.
- Symptoms include a complaint of 'pseudoclaudication' and deep tendon reflex responses are hyporeflexic or absent. Table 6.3

Table 6.3 Nerve root damage

NERVE ROOT	SENSORY DEFICIT	MOTOR DEFICIT	DEEP TENDON REFLEX RESPONSE
4th lumbar	Medial lower leg Medial malleolus Medial foot	Quadriceps femoris	Diminished patellar Normal Achilles
5th lumbar	Anterolateral lower leg Dorsal foot	Extensor hallucis longus	Normal patellar Normal Achilles
1st sacral	Posterolateral lower leg	Triceps surae Plantar foot	Normal patellar Diminished Achilles

Cerebellar lesions

- Cerebellar pathology in the lower extremity is recognised by classic, unco-ordinated ataxic gait.
- Voluntary movements cannot be performed smoothly.
- Cerebellar gait is recognised as a wide-based gait with a slow, jerky and irregular cadence.
- *Friedreich's ataxia* is also known as hereditary spinocerebellar ataxia:
  - it is an autosomal recessive gene defect carried on the pericentric region of chromosome 9
  - it is characterised by the progressive loss of voluntary muscle co-ordination, obstructive cardiac hypertrophy and the possibility of diabetes mellitus
  - symptoms begin between the ages of 5 and 15 years
  - early loss of vibratory and position sense
  - loss of the Achilles and patellar deep tendon reflex responses and a positive Babinski sign
  - patients may have a tendency to stagger and fall
  - weakness is greatest in the peroneal muscle group resulting in a cavus foot type with flexion contracture of the digits
  - gait is unsteady with a wide base, characteristics of basal ganglia lesions.

Hyperkinetic dyskinesias

- Huntington's chorea is transmitted by autosomal dominant inheritance and is characterised by choreic involuntary movement, progressive dementia and psychiatric and behavioural disturbances.
- Sydenham's chorea or St Vitus' dance:
  - sydenham's chorea is more common in girls
  - the condition may first be recognised by the presence of facial grimacing slowly progressing to involuntary flinging movements and sudden jerks which may be more prevalent in the upper extremities.

Hypokinetic dyskinesias

Parkinsonism

- Parkinsonism is a distinctive symptom complex characterised by tremor, muscular rigidity, bradykinesia and characteristic alterations of posture and attitude of the extremities and is sometimes referred to as paralysis agitans.
- Clinical features include tremor, rigidity, bradykinesia and disturbances in gait and posture.
- A resting, 'pill-rolling' tremor is common.
- The patient acquires a stooped posture with the head tilted forward, arms flexed at the wrists and elbows and walks with a shuffling gait.
- There is loss of facial expression early in the disease leading to monotonous, stuttering and 'deliberate' speech patterns.
- Patients with advanced disease present with a classic shuffling gait.

Cerebral palsy

- A chronic, non-progressive disorder affecting motor dysfunction
- Evident in the second year of life

Table 6.4 Cerebral palsy

TYPE OF CEREBRAL PALSY	AREA OF INJURY	CLINICAL INVOLVEMENT
Spastic: 50–70%	Motor cortex lesion	
Monoplegia	One limb involved affected	Spastic movement of arm or leg
Diplegia/paraplegia	Two limbs involved	Spastic movement of arms or legs
Quadriplegia	Four limbs involved	Spastic movement of all four limbs
Hemiplegia	One side affected	Ipsilateral involvement of arm and leg
Double hemiplegia	Both sides	Spastic movement is not symmetrical
Athetoid: 10–20%	Basal ganglia lesion	Uncontrolled, unco-ordinated movements
Ataxic: 5–10%	Cerebellar lesion	Inco-ordination of movement or balance
Mixed: 10%	Combination of lesions	Spastic/athetoid most common

- Early clinical signs include a change in muscle tone, asymmetry of movement where there is greater involvement of one side or limb and delay in sitting up, crawling and walking
- The spastic limbs are usually thinner and smaller with hyper-reflexia and clonus
- The Babinski sign is usually present in postnatal cases. Internal hip rotation; involvement of the knee flexors and plantar extensors results in toe walking and a cavo-varus foot deformity
- Arms are held adducted at the shoulders and flexed at the elbows and wrists
- Patients demonstrate a 'scissored' gait. Table 6.4

The classifications include:

- *athetotic cerebral palsy* – characterised by slow, uncontrolled, writhing movements which may be continuous or intermittent:
  - there is a slow, serpentine movement of the arms and legs interposed upon postures of flexion with supination and extension with pronation accompanied by rotatory movements of the neck
- *ataxic cerebral palsy* occurs secondary to cerebellar dysfunction and is characterised by an inability to control the rate, range, direction and force of fine motor movements:
  - there is a wide base of gait
- *mixed cerebral palsy* is a combination of spastic and athetotic movements.

AUTONOMIC NERVOUS SYSTEM

Sympathetic nervous system dysfunction in the lower extremity

- Overactivity results in vasoconstriction and hyperhidrosis resulting in a cyanotic-appearing, cool, clammy extremity
- Underactivity or a lack of sympathetic regulation causes vasodilation and anhidrosis identified by the presence of bounding pulses, erythema and significant xerosis
- *Hyperhidrosis* represents increased activity of the sympathetic nervous system
- *Raynaud's disease* occurs most frequently in women between the ages of 18 and 40 years:
  - when associated with many collagen vascular diseases, it is referred to as Raynaud's phenomenon
  - Raynaud's disease is characterised by a 'triphasic' colour response of pallor, cyanosis and rubor
- *Acrocyanosis* occurs secondary to an overactive sympathetic nervous system, aetiology unknown:
  - it is characterised by patchy cyanosis at the distal portions of the extremities
  - differentiated from Raynaud's disease by the persistence of cyanosis
  - symptoms include swelling, decreased touch, heat, cold and pain perception, paraesthesias and hyperhidrosis
- *Familial dysautonomia* is also known as Riley–Day syndrome and is characterised by a complete indifference to pain. It is inherited as an autosomal recessive trait and occurs in individuals of Mediterranean descent:
  - the most distinctive clinical feature is the absence of tears with emotional crying
  - a cavus foot type and the presence of trophic ulcers are frequent findings in the lower extremity
- *Reflex sympathetic dystrophy* was renamed complex regional pain syndrome type I: Fig 6.7
  - it is believed to occur as a secondary vasomotor instability in some way mediated by the sympathetic nervous system
  - frequently associated with a minor form of trauma such as sprains, soft-tissue wounds, fractures of varied severity, surgical procedures and infection, there is no obvious nerve lesion
  - causalgia was renamed complex regional pain syndrome type II and is characterised by the same clinical presentation; however, there is an identifiable nerve injury
  - sympathetically maintained pain is an additional classification of this type of injury and is characterised as pain restricted to the distribution of a single nerve
  - the key finding in all these syndromes is pain out of proportion to the severity of the injury.

Diabetic peripheral neuropathy

- Distal symmetrical polyneuropathy is the most common type of neuropathy in diabetics.
- Patients present with prominent paraesthesias and autonomic nervous system dysfunction recognised by the presence of orthostatic hypotension, resting tachycardia and distal anhidrosis.

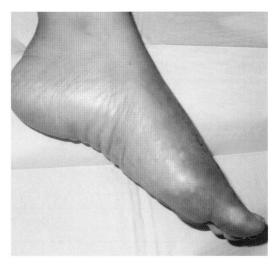

Figure 6.7 Complex regional pain syndrome. Mottled cyanosis with oedema in a 31-year-old female 3 weeks following surgical correction of a bunion deformity. Symptoms were brought on abruptly by placing the foot in a dependent position.

Table 6.5 Modified classification system of Eichenholtz

STAGE	RADIOGRAPHIC FINDINGS
0 Clinical	Erythema, oedema and increased temperature
I Development	Generalised demineralisation Periarticular fragmentation Loose body formation Joint dislocation
II Coalescence	Organisation and early healing of fracture fragments Periosteal new bone formation Resorption of bony debris
III Reconstruction or consolidation	Greater definition of bony contours Reconstruction or ankylosis of involved bones

- Symptoms of large-fibre involvement include tingling, burning, numbness, allodynia or deep lancinating pain.
- Sensory ataxia may occur as a result of diminished vibratory and proprioceptive sense. Sensory changes do not always correlate with nerve conduction deficits.
- Deep tendon reflex responses are attenuated or absent and there may be distal motor weakness.
- Progression of nerve injury leads to the loss of ability to detect small objects or stimuli resulting ultimately in the neurotrophic or insensate diabetic foot. This is the cause of diabetic ulceration in up to 85% of patients.

Table 6.6 Clinical features of hypertrophic Charcot joint disease

VASCULAR	NEUROPATHIC	SKELETAL	CUTANEOUS SEQUELAE
Bounding pulses	Diminished or absent	'Rocker bottom' foot	Hyperkeratosis
Erythema	Pain and vibratory sense	Midfoot subluxations	Neurotrophic ulceration
Oedema	Proprioception	Digital contractures	Secondary infection
Warmth	Deep tendon reflexes	Hypermobility	

Table 6.7 Damage to upper and lower motor neuron lesions

MOTOR UPPER NEURON LESION	LOWER MOTOR NEURON LESION
Spastic paralysis	Flaccid paralysis
Hyper-reflexia	Hyporeflexia
Babinski sign present	Babinski sign absent
No fasciculations or fibrillations	Fasciculations and fibrillations

Charcot joint disease

- Charcot joint disease is also referred to as neuropathic osteoarthropathy.
- There are two forms: atrophic and hypertrophic.
- Atrophic joint disease occurs much less frequently. It may be referred to as diabetic osteolysis and is a form of bone resorption thought to be brought on by hyperaemia.
- It is generally localised to the forefoot. Table 6.5
- Hypertrophic Charcot joint disease is most likely multifactorial.
- Hypertrophic Charcot joint disease usually occurs at the midfoot, rearfoot or ankle. Table 6.6, Table 6.7

Chapter | **7** |

Podiatry in the management of Hansen's disease (leprosy) and tropical diseases

HANSEN'S DISEASE

Hansen's disease (HD), or hanseniasis, are the preferred terms for leprosy as they do not have the same connotations that the term leprosy does.

Epidemiology (see Table 7.1)

- Hansen's disease is essentially a problem in the developing countries. The prevalence figures only suggest the number of people registered for treatment and do not give any indication of those who are 'cured' but remain permanently impaired. Figures for the total number of affected people are not available but could be in the region of millions.
- After diabetes mellitus, HD is the most common cause of sensory neuropathy globally and is probably the major cause of neuropathy in Asia and Africa, where it affects predominantly the lower socio-economic groups.
- Aerosol contamination remains the most likely form of transmission and there is evidence which demonstrates that infected droplets can be expelled during sneezing, coughing and even talking. Droplets may also be absorbed by dust, and viable *M. leprae* has been identified in desiccated secretions a week after expectorating.
- The bacillus is not virulent; infected subjects can host vast numbers without feeling any ill effect, and chemotherapy rapidly compromises the viability of the bacillus. It is, therefore, from undiagnosed, multibacillary hosts that the threat of infection is greatest.

Classification

- The Ridley–Jopling classification describes the spectrum of disease from tuberculoid (TT), which demonstrates vigorous resistance and low infection (paucibacillary, PB), to lepromatous (LL), which demonstrates severely compromised resistance and massive infection (multibacillary, MB). Borderline (BB) describes resistance that lies between the two polar responses.

- Neuropathy in tuberculoid leprosy:
  - the most significant changes in tuberculoid leprosy involve the cutaneous and subcutaneous nerves. Nerve damage is an inherent effect of host response and is not related to massive proliferation of bacilli. Infected nerves are invaded and destroyed beyond recognition by epithelioid granulomae.
  - the most frequently affected nerves in the lower limb are the common peroneal and the posterior tibial nerves. The saphenous and the sural nerves are less commonly affected.
- Neuropathy in lepromatous leprosy:
  - due to depressed cell-mediated immunity in lepromatous leprosy, the haematogenous spread of the bacilli allows the unchecked proliferation of bacilli. Nerve damage is slower to become apparent than in other forms of leprosy. It is these cells that are known as lepra cells, carrying masses of bacilli collectively called globi.
  - symmetrical and bilateral sensory loss of lepromatous leprosy is explained by the massive and widespread distribution of bacilli. The sites of nerve lesions appear to be related to body temperature.
- Neuropathy in borderline (dimorphous) leprosy:
  - while nerve damage in borderline leprosy is essentially limited to the same sites as those common in lepromatous leprosy, the potential for uncharacteristic neurological defects is greater. Cases of borderline leprosy demonstrate the greatest potential for catastrophic peripheral nerve damage. This is explained by a dual effect.
  - where a borderline case demonstrates a tendency to fall closer to the tuberculoid pole (BT), paralysis and sensory loss are always asymmetrical. Where borderline cases lie at the midpoint of the spectrum (BB), involvement is asymmetrical and indicates intracutaneous nerve dysfunction because the borders of insensitivity do not conform to dermatomes. In a low-resistance borderline case (BL) there will be numerous lesions, symmetrically distributed. Areas of insensitivity may exceed the borders of lesions, and temperature-linked patterns of sensory loss become apparent.

The lower limb in Hansen's disease

Anaesthesia

The high density of Vater–Pacini corpuscles in the subcutaneous fat chambers provides an acute sense of deep pressure and vibration. These modalities are associated with high-frequency shock and tissue displacement, whereas it is postulated that the Meissener's corpuscles register low-frequency shock. The dual effect of these modalities is that the foot's movement against the ground and the character of the weight-bearing surface may be perceived.

Factors associated with plantar ulceration

- Motor paralysis – It has been suggested that only 6% of ulcerated feet display anaesthesia alone; when the foot was further compromised by intrinsic muscular paralysis this figure was increased 10-fold. It is probable that paralysis of the intrinsic muscles increases the vulnerability of the foot by creating instability during propulsion. The extent to which pre-existing functional abnormalities could exacerbate this condition has not been widely considered:
  - *claw toe* deformity is a common feature of the neuropathic foot in Hansen's disease and is generally considered to indicate intrinsic muscle paralysis.

- *extrinsic muscle paralysis. M. leprae* appears to have a predilection for cooler sites such as the peroneal nerve as it winds around the fibular neck. Peroneal and anterior compartment paralysis is not uncommon. The resulting foot drop deformity can severely compromise an affected person. Excessive lateral and forefoot loading predisposes the patient to ulceration, particularly under the 5th metatarsal head.
- Pre-existing pathomechanical foot function – Of initial ulcers that occur on the forefoot, the most common sites are: on the plantar aspect of the proximal phalanx of the hallux, the 2nd metatarsal head and the area between the 1st metatarsal head and the proximal phalanx of the hallux.
- Tarsal disintegration – In late lepromatous leprosy, a complication may be the massive infiltration of bacilli into the bones of the foot, which can result in fracture and disintegration of tarsal bones.
- Absorption and pathological fractures – Active secondary infection of ulceration may lead to periostitis and osteomyelitis, which commonly leads to sequestration. Hyperaemia, associated with chronic plantar ulceration, and active infection of bone can also cause osteoporosis and predisposes it to pathological fractures, particularly when pain sensation in the joints is lost.
- Autonomic impairment – The impairment of dermal sympathetic nerve function may result in the loss of sweat and axon reflexes.
- Social and behavioural factors.

Complications of ulceration

- Secondary infection – Common causative organisms implicated are *Staphylococcus aureus, Streptococcus haemolyticas, Pseudomonas aeruginosa, Proteus mirabilis* and *Escherichia coli*. Infection spreads rapidly along tendon sheaths and into synovial joint spaces. Infective arthritis and osteomyeltis are common sequelae.
- Squamous cell carcinoma – Hyperplasia, influenced by chronic irritation, initiates the regeneration of cells which manifest as papillomatoses adapted to irritation. Continued irritation leads to dysplasia with decreasing cell differentiation and, ultimately, carcinoma.

Treatment of pedal pathologies

Table 7.1 Countries with the highest prevalence rates in 1998 (WHO 1999)			
COUNTRIES	PREVALENCE	PREVALENCE PER 10000	NEW CASE DETECTION RATE RATE
India	527 344	5.3	53.16
Brazil	72 953	4.33	25.86
Indonesia	29 225	1.41	7.42
Myanmar	13 581	2.74	18.35
Bangladesh	13 248	1.03	8.80

Continued

Table 7.1 Countries with the highest prevalence rates in 1998 (WHO 1999)—cont'd

COUNTRIES	PREVALENCE	PREVALENCE PER 10000	NEW CASE DETECTION RATE RATE
Nigeria	12 878	1.06	5.89
Nepal	12 540	5.30	31.49
Mozambique	11 072	6.24	23.64
Madagascar	11 005	6.78	71.23
Philippines	8 749	1.22	6.89

TROPICAL DISEASES

- Skin infection and tropical diseases presenting on the foot may represent a primary condition or a secondary manifestation of illness elsewhere in the body. Cutaneous larva migrans, madura foot, and localised cutaneous simple leishmaniasis are examples of the former, whereas the latter can be exemplified by systemic conditions such as leprosy, disseminated leishmaniasis and coccidioidomycosis.
- The identification of extracutaneous signs such as fever, enlarged lymph nodes, and general malaise indicate systemic illness, and these findings should prompt immediate action for an appropriate referral.
- The prevalence of skin diseases in the tropics is similar to that found in developed countries. The main differences found in tropical settings are a higher incidence of endemic infectious diseases, a lower frequency of skin malignancy, and the lack or decreased availability of podiatric and dermatological services.

Bacterial infections

Pyogenic infections

Aetiology and pathogenesis

- Common bacterial infections of the skin are caused by *Staphylococcus* and *Streptococcus* species. The port of entry for these pathogenic organisms is often unnoticed by both the patient and doctor, but minor injuries, insect bites, friction blisters, or superficial fungal infection are the commonest found in clinical practice.

Clinical findings and diagnosis

- The clinical spectrum of pyogenic infections of the foot includes folliculitis, furuncle and carbuncle formation on areas with hair follicles. Plaques of impetigo and infiltrated thickened dermis can affect any region of the foot, and are respectively caused by *Staphylococcus* and *Streptococcus* species. Abscess formation, cellulitis, and necrotic ulceration represent the more severe end of the spectrum.

- The perimalleolar regions are far more commonly affected than other areas of the foot as they are exposed to mechanical trauma. The dorsum, toes and heels follow in frequency.
- Common clinical signs of pyogenic infections include a variety of manifestations such as erythema, inflammation, pus discharge, abscess formation, ulceration, blistering, necrotising lesions and gangrene.

Management and treatment

- Mild infections are successfully treated with bathing or soaking the affected foot in potassium permanganate solution (1 : 10 000 dilution in water) for 15 minutes daily. Other mild superficial infections, such as isolated plaques of impetigo or impetiginised eczema, respond well to antiseptic or antimicrobial creams and ointments containing cetrimide, chlorhexidine, fucidic acid or mupirocin.
- Acute or chronic foot eczema requires treatment with potent topical steroids in order to eliminate risk factors for infection. Infections with multiple lesions, or those involving larger areas of the foot, require a complete course of systemic β-lactam or macrolide antibiotics in addition to the above topical treatments.
- Recurrent episodes of cellulitis require longer courses of these antibiotics, and hospitalisation followed by surgical debridement is mandatory in necrotic lesions, gangrenous plaques, and deeper infections with severe fasciitis. Superficial infections of the foot skin complicated by deeper involvement with necrosis of soft tissues carry a high mortality rate of up to 25%.

Treponemal infections

- Cosmopolitan treponemal diseases such as secondary *syphilis* present with an asymptomatic, symmetrical papular eruption and scaling of plantar regions. Other clinical features, such as concurrent palmar involvement, the history of a primary chancre, and the characteristic trunkal rash, confirm the clinical suspicion.
- *Yaws* is a treponemal tropical disease manifesting on the feet and periorificial skin on the face. Late tertiary infection results in asymptomatic palmoplantar keratoderma that develops nodular hyperkeratotic lesions leading to painful disability; hence the characteristic walk known as 'crab yaws'.
- Tropical sea-borne infections by halophilic *Vibrio vulnificus* can produce localised or systemic disease manifested by acute and painful erythema, purpura, oedema and necrosis on one or both feet. The infection is acquired by direct traumatic inoculation in estuaries and seawater, or by ingestion of raw seafood, particularly oysters.
- Exfoliation of the plantar skin is part of the complex and severe picture in cosmopolitan cases with *staphylococcal scalded skin syndrome* (SSSS).
- Necrotic ulceration of the foot can result from tropical *cutaneous diphtheria* caused by *Corynebacterium diphtheriae*. Cutaneous diphtheria commonly manifests as a non-healing single ulcerated lesion on the toe or toe cleft lasting between 4 and 12 weeks.

Mycobacterial infections

- Several mycobacterial species can cause primary or secondary infection of the foot. The 'swimming' or 'fish tank granuloma' is an infection caused by

Mycobacterium marinum. Other common chronic mycobacterial tropical infections include leprosy, tuberculosis, and Buruli ulcer. These are respectively caused by *M. leprae*, *M. tuberculosis*, and *M. ulcerans*.

- Mycobacterial skin diseases can be acquired by direct skin contact with a patient, by direct accidental or occupational inoculation, and by inhalation of the infective organisms. Particular clinical forms of cutaneous tuberculosis result following haematogenous dissemination from a primary infection elsewhere. The respiratory route is particularly important for Hansen's disease and diverse forms of pulmonary tuberculosis.

- In the case of Buruli ulcer it has recently been suggested that contact with infected water in rural areas of Africa may represent the main source of infection.

Clinical findings and diagnosis

- Fish-tank granuloma affects more commonly the fingers or hand but it has also been described on the foot. The disease manifests as a localised progressing swelling with variable pain, and the appearance, within a few weeks, of nodular or verrucous skin lesions on the affected area. These lesions can show ulceration and bleeding from the disease process itself but also from mechanical trauma. The dorsal aspects of the foot and the malleolar regions are exposed to trauma and, therefore, direct inoculation commonly takes place on these regions.

- Hansen's disease is a chronic disease that affects not only the skin of one foot or both feet, but also particularly the peripheral nerves bilaterally. The foot is one of the anatomical sites where inflammation, characteristic skin lesions, and nerve damage occur in the course of the disease. The commonest lesions affecting one or both feet are nodules, erythematous plaques, or hypopigmented patches. Mutilating lesions of the toes result from bone resorption, mechanical trauma and secondary bacterial infection.

- Skin tuberculosis affects individuals of all ages and both sexes who present with a wide variety of clinical pictures that frequently affect the lower limbs and particularly one foot or both feet. However, lupus vulgaris and papulonecrotic tuberculide are more common in females, whereas tuberculosis verrucosa cutis is rare in children. By far the main clinical presentation of cutaneous tuberculosis affecting the adult foot is tuberculosis verrucosa cutis. Commonly observed asymptomatic lesions include dry patches of atrophic skin, pigmentary changes, nodules, and plaques of verrucous lesions. The total plaque of tuberculosis can measure between 2 and 12 cm in diameter, but chronic and larger lesions can involve most of the foot dorsum and lateral aspects.

- Buruli ulcer affects mainly young individuals in rural Africa – particularly in West Africa, where an increase in incidence has been reported. More than two-thirds of the cases present in children below the age of 15. Lesions present as papules or small nodules that slowly increase in size to the point of causing an area of inflammation and, subsequently, ulceration of the skin with undermined edges. Active indolent phagedenism manifests, often involving large areas of the affected limb.

- Oedematous forms may progress rapidly and cause a panniculitis with destruction of underlying tissues such as fascia and bone. In cases where a large ulceration is followed by healing, contractures of the affected limb result from scarring. Severe scarring and contractures have been identified as a high morbidity factor for disability and up to 10% require amputation of the deformed limb.

Management and treatment

- Most mycobacterial diseases affecting the skin represent a public health priority, not only for the endemic countries, but also at an international level, as established by the World Health Organization (WHO). Mycobacteria are known to develop resistance to antibiotics and it is imperative that all cases be treated with combinations of at least two drugs. The main drugs with anti-mycobacterial activity are rifampin, ethambutol, pirazinamide, clofazimine, sulfone, isoniazide, macrolide antibiotics, tetracyclines and quinolones. Early lesions of fish-tank granuloma, skin tuberculosis and, in particular, those caused by Buruli ulcer, require surgical excision.

Bacterial mycetoma

- *Nocardia*, *Actinomadura* and *Streptomyces* species are the common aetiological agents of 'madura foot' or actinomycetoma. This form of bacterial mycetoma occurs in tropical countries and the main case series have been reported from Sudan, Senegal, Nigeria, Saudi Arabia, India and Mexico. The infection is acquired by direct inoculation of bacteria into the skin.

Clinical findings and diagnosis

- The disease is characterised by a chronic course with inflammation, formation of sinus tracts discharging 'grains' and progressive deformity of the affected foot. Healing of discharging sinus tracts throughout years determines scarring with atrophic skin plaques and secondary pigmentary changes.
- The main differential diagnosis includes mycetoma caused by fungi (see Eumycetoma, p. 124), but other forms of 'cold' abscess formation, histoplasmosis, chromoblastomycosis, cutaneous tuberculosis and sarcoidosis are the other main conditions to consider. Direct microscopy to disclose the 'grains' discharged from sinus tracts confirms the diagnosis and the culture of this material also provides a definite diagnosis of actinomycetoma.

Parasitic diseases, ectoparasite infestations and bites

Cutaneous larva migrans

This dermatosis results from the accidental penetration of the human skin by parasitic larvae from domestic canine and feline hosts.

- The plantar regions of one foot or both feet represent the main anatomical site affected by cutaneous larva migrans, but any part of the body in contact with infested soil or sand can be involved. Individuals of all age groups and both sexes can be affected and the disease is a common problem for tourists on beach holidays where they walk on bare feet or lay on the infested sand. It is variable in severity, but most commonly intense pruritus and burning sensation are the main symptoms.

Leishmaniasis

- *Leishmania* species parasites are protozoan organisms transmitted to humans and other vertebrates by the bite of female sandflies. Most *Leishmania* species can cause skin or mucocutaneous disease, but a few of them affect internal organs as well. The bite of the sandfly commonly targets exposed areas such as the external ankles during walking or else medial regions of the foot when the host is at rest.

- Several drugs are effective against *Leishmania* parasites and these include: pentavalent antimonials, amphotericin B, triazole and alylamine antifungal compounds. However, the only treatment of choice for a number of species is the intravenous administration of antimonials carefully monitored in hospital and administered only by experienced personnel.

Tungiasis

- A localised skin disease commonly affecting one foot and caused by the burrowing flea *Tunga penetrans*. This is also known as chigoe infestation, jigger, sandflea, chigoe and puce chique (Fr). The fleas commonly affect one foot, penetrating the soft skin on the toe web spaces, but other areas of toes and plantar aspects on the foot can be affected.
- Curettage, cryotherapy, surgical excision or careful removal of the flea and eggs are the potential treatments.

Scabies

- Poor tropical countries with low standards of hygiene and, particularly, overcrowding suffer from cyclical outbreaks of severe and chronic forms. The human scabies mite *Sarcoptes scabiei* commonly affects the skin of both feet of infants and children.
- It appears as papules with or without excoriation, and S-shaped burrows. Infants and young children present with papular, vesicular, and/or nodular lesions on both plantar regions but other parts of the feet can be affected.
- Topical treatment overnight with benzyl benzoate, malathion, lindane or permethrine, lotion or cream, is usually effective.

Ticks

- Ectoparasites capable of transmitting severe viral, rickettsial, bacterial and parasitic diseases. Soft ticks of the Argasidae family are more prevalent in the tropics and subtropical regions of the world and transmit agents of tick-borne relapsing fever.
- Removal of the tick can be carried out by applying a tight dressing or cloth impregnated with chloroform, petrol, or ether onto the tick body. The organism is carefully removed a few minutes later, avoiding the rupture of head and mouth-parts that can be left behind in the skin.

Fleas

- Fleas bite humans in order to get a blood meal and in doing so produce a localised inflammatory reaction which appears as prurigo with papules, vesicles or small nodules. Both feet and lower legs are characteristic and the lesions are often found in clusters.

Fungal conditions

Eumycetoma

- *Madurella mycetomatis*, *Pseudoallescheria boydii* and *Leptosphaeria senegalensis* are the main aetiological agents of true fungal mycetoma, also known as eumycetoma. A generic term, 'Madura foot' is currently used to describe all forms of bacterial and fungal mycetoma.

- It affects predominantly young male individuals between 20 and 50 years of age. The perimalleolar region and the dorsum are the most commonly affected sites. The characteristic clinical signs include a nodule or irregular swelling followed by sinus tract formation and discharge of purulent material containing the characteristic grains.
- Systemic antibiotics in combination, such as streptomycin, cotrimoxazol, amikacin, dapsone and rifampin, are the drugs of choice that require long-term administration.

Chromoblastomycosis

- Chromoblastomycosis is a chronic infection caused by fungi of the genera *Fonsecaea, Cladosporium* and *Phialophora*. The commonest site affected in sporadic infections is the foot, and the chronic verrucous plaque appears on the dorsum or the perimalleolar region.
- It is accepted that chromoblastomycosis is not easy to treat medically, and patients require long-term treatment. Localised and early cases respond successfully to complete surgical excision of the lesion, and thermosurgery has also been reported to be of benefit.

Dermatophytes (see Chapter 16 Tinea Pedis)

Viral infections

- Viral infections with foot involvement that are prevalent in the tropics include plantar warts, Kaposi's sarcoma, and severe blistering forms by varicella.

Miscellaneous conditions

- Ainhum – This uncommon condition affecting the fifth toe of adults in tropical Africa is also called spontaneous dactylolysis. A painful constricting band of fibrotic tissue results in spontaneous amputation of the toe.
- Pellagra is caused by a nutritional deficiency of niacin and manifests with the triad dermatitis, diarrhoea and dementia (3Ds). Clinically, it manifests with a remarkable photosensitive rash that may show an eczematoid pattern with hyperpigmentation affecting the face, neck and both lower limbs, which present with signs similar to those found in stasis dermatitis. Eczematoid changes, xerosis and hyperpigmented patches are present symmetrically on both feet.
- Sea-borne conditions present following contact or traumatic skin injury from jelly fish, coral, anemones, sea-urchins and venomous fish. A variety of acute clinical pictures manifest as contact eczema, stings, burns and penetrating injuries, whereas vasoactive phenomena represent the common pathogenic mechanism in direct skin poisoning.

Chapter | **8** |

Musculoskeletal disorders

INTRODUCTION

Rheumatology practice covers a heterogeneous range of more than 200 disorders with varied aetiologies, which affect joints, bones, muscles and soft tissues, and have a variety of systemic features. However, their common feature is their effect on the musculoskeletal system.

Epidemiology

- 1 : 7 adults
- 1 : 20 severe musculoskeletal disorders
- Prevalence increases steadily with age, and by the age of 75 years as high as 1 : 3
- Impact on quality of life increases as the number of affected sites increases.

Disability pathway

See Fig 8.1.

Management generally

- Classical approach – slowly escalating drug therapy
- Classical approach has been superseded by a new paradigm of early and aggressive treatment, and combination therapies using disease-modifying anti-rheumatic drugs (DMARDs)
- See Fig 8.2 for schemata of medical management
- Early management is aggressive, and combinations of DMARDs are used to suppress inflammation nearer to disease onset, so limiting irreversible joint damage
- In inflammatory arthritis the goal is to establish and maintain disease remission, non-steroidal anti-inflammatory drugs (NSAIDs) (ibuprofen, diclofenac, indometacin or cyclo-oxygenase-2 (cox-2) inhibitors according to risk factors), provide immediate reduction in pain and stiffness:
  - DMARD therapy within 3 months of disease onset is highly effective in controlling immune-mediated inflammatory disease (IMIDs)

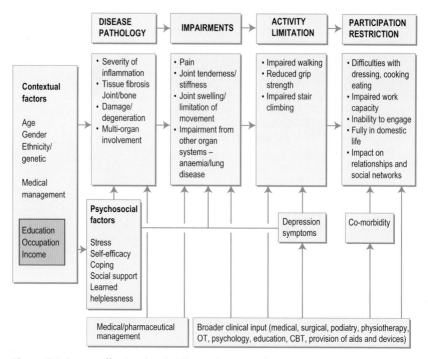

Figure 8.1 Factors affecting the disability pathway in inflammatory arthritis. *From the original concept proposed by Nagi (1965) and modified by Escolante (2002), adapted here to incorporate WHO ICF definitions.*

(methotrexate, hydroxychloroquine, with sulfasalazine becoming increasingly marginalised, and Leflunomide – new drug)

- the new, biologic DMARDs inhibit cytokine activity high up in the inflammatory pathway. Most common 'biologics' are the agents active against tumour necrosis factor α (TNF α); etanercept (Enbrel), infliximab (Remicade) and adalimumab (Humira).

THE FOOT IN RHEUMATOLOGY

There is no validated, standardised assessment for the foot in musculoskeletal conditions.

Preferred protocol – Look-Feel-Move.

History

- Clerking information
- Demographics
- General medical history – including (as appropriate) duration of disease, medications, disease activity markers
- Presenting complaint – history and documentation including pain maps and patient-completed baseline health outcome measures (MFPDQ, FFI, LFIS – *see outcomes section*).

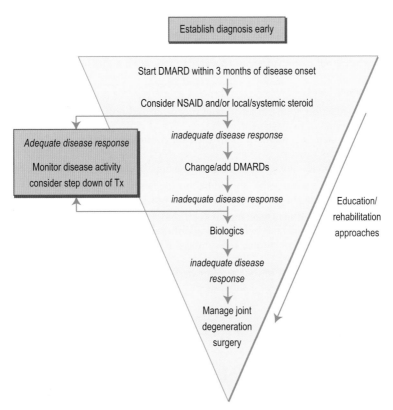

Figure 8.2 An abridged schema for the medical management of RA *(adapted from ACR guidelines 2002).*

Observation (non-weight bearing)

- Musculoskeletal system/disease state:
  - limb alignment
  - joint/soft tissue swellings
  - dermal signs
- Presenting complaint:
  - visible lesions measured and dimensions recorded
  - recording of tender and swollen joints counts are on a Ritchie-type chart
- Footwear assessment – suitability, wear patterns, distortion of uppers.

Observation (weight bearing)

- Limb alignment – large joint and limb segment alignment, foot posture in quiet standing (supplemented with photographic images as appropriate)
- Comparison of weight-bearing observations with non-weight-bearing
- Observation of gait.

Examination

- Provocation/reproduction of pain/symptoms – palpation, active motion, passive motion
- Systematic palpation and movement of structures moving from proximal to distal – bony structures, joints, soft tissues

- Plain X-ray is usually still the imaging modality of first choice
- High-resolution ultrasound (HRUS) is becoming increasingly popular as a 'bedside' modality in rheumatology as it is low risk, differentiates soft-tissue structures well and involves no exposure to ionisation radiation.

Foot management

- Callus reduction, footwear advice and provision, and orthosis prescription are mainstays of management
- Injectable steroid is useful in many cases for controlling local areas of inflammatory activity
- Multidisciplinary care is important in managing rheumatology patients.

The foot health services that should be provided as part of a multidisciplinary foot-health team in rheumatology fall into five categories:

- education and self-management advice, including on footwear
- provision of, or assistance with, finding orthoses and footwear
- general foot care, nail cutting, corn and callus reduction, provision of padding
- high-risk management of the vasculitic or ulcerative foot
- extended scope practice and surgery.

SPECIFIC DISEASES

Seropositive inflammatory arthritis

Rheumatoid arthritis

Definition

Rheumatoid arthritis (RA) is a chronic, immune-mediated inflammatory disease with polyarthritis as its main feature. Prevalence of RA in the population is approximately 7.7 per thousand (0.8%). Average age at onset was 55 years. Ratio 3 : 1 females : males.

Diagnosis is made according to diagnostic criteria defined by the American College of Rheumatology (Box 8.1); however, consensus-based referral recommendations for primary care practitioners suggest inflammatory (rheumatoid) arthritis should be considered, and patients referred rapidly for a rheumatology opinion if they demonstrate:

Box 8.1 **1987 ACR Criteria for the diagnosis of rheumatoid arthritis**

Four or more must be present from:

1. Morning stiffness for at least 1 hour, and present for at least 6 weeks
2. Swelling of three or more joints for at least 6 weeks
3. Swelling of the wrist, metacarpophalangeal or proximal interphalangeal joints for 6 or more weeks
4. Symmetric joint swelling
5. Hand radiograph changes typical of rheumatoid arthritis that must include erosions or unequivocal bony decalcification
6. Rheumatoid nodules
7. Serum rheumatoid factor by a method positive in less than 5% of normals.

- three or more swollen joints
- pain on lateral compression of the metacarpo- or metatarso-phalangeal joints (a positive squeeze test)
- morning stiffness of ≥30 minutes duration.

Histopathology

Underlying histopathology is of:

- an immune-mediated synovitis caused by a faulty auto-immune response to proteins such as immunoglobulin G
- hyperplasic synovial membrane of the affected joint, infiltrated with inflammatory cells which promote secretion of pro-inflammatory cytokines
- synovial membrane proliferating further forming a pannus, which increasingly intrudes into the joint space
- pannus releasing enzymes that degrade cartilage and the connective tissue matrix.

The prevalence and impact of foot problems is related to disease duration and the foot is affected eventually in nearly all people with RA, usually in a symmetrical pattern:

- joint pain and stiffness most common initial presentation
- range of other features may also be found including tenosynovitis, nodule formation, and tarsal tunnel syndrome, reflecting the widespread soft tissue involvement
- retrocalcaneal bursitis is common, and often coexists with inflammation of the tendo Achilles, and long flexor and extensor tendon sheaths
- spurs can be found on the plantar surface of the calcaneus, posterior spurs at the insertion of the tendo Achilles tend to be smaller and are often asymptomatic
- ankle (talocrural) joint degeneration occurs relatively rarely in RA and is confined to severe and late-stage disease
- ankle joint change is almost always preceded by subtalar joint (STJ) involvement
- synovitis in the hindfoot joints leads to systematic alterations in hindfoot structure and function
- altered function, combined with the effect of load-bearing and increased soft-tissue laxity, lead the hindfoot to function in a progressively more pronated position, with the heel becoming more inclined into valgus and the tibia more internally rotated
- initially the deformities are largely reducible, and the elastic response of the soft tissues allows for correction
- rigid functional orthoses have been shown to restore normal function, and to slow the progression of fixed deformity
- in the valgus rheumatoid foot, synovitis and compression of tissues on the medial aspect of the hindfoot can lead to tarsal tunnel syndrome – paraesthesia/burning sensation over the distribution of the tibial nerve on the plantar surface of the foot
- tarsal tunnel syndrome may respond to local injection of corticosteroid, but may require surgical decompression
- where significant deformity adaptive footwear might be necessary
- addition of external flanges to the heel along with reinforcement of the heel counter and medial arch of the upper of the shoes can aid with hindfoot stability
- extra depth shoes allow for an orthosis

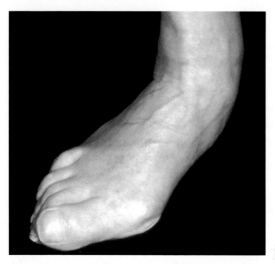

Figure 8.3 The clinical appearance of the forefoot deformity typical of RA.

- joints of the midfoot are affected widely, with the talo-navicular joint, and Lisfranc's joints affected
- metatarsophalangeal joints (MTPJs) are the joints most commonly affected – symmetrical distribution
- synovitis can lead to swelling of the digits, and MTPJ synovitis, noted clinically as a warm boggy feeling to the joint on palpation
- can lead to separation of neighbouring toes (the so-called 'daylight sign')
- rheumatoid forefoot will develop a typical marked hallux valgus type presentation and hammer toe deformities of the lesser toes Fig 8.3
- prominent adventitious bursae develop under the metatarsal heads and these are frequently overlaid with callus
- plantar pressure data show the areas of increased pressure to be highly localised and patients often describe a feeling of 'walking on pebbles'
- gait velocity decreases as both cadence and stride length are reduced
- the double support period extends to minimise the forces applied to the foot, and a reluctance to load the forefoot leads to delay in loading and alteration of the velocity of centre of pressure profile
- accommodative footwear can be provided off-the-shelf if the requirement is simply for extra depth or soft uppers in the toe box
- patients own shoes may be adapted in some cases, or bespoke shoes may still be made
- soft flexible uppers made of soft leathers or stretchable textile can be very helpful in reducing the pressure on deformed digits (Fig 8.4), and in accommodating the increased width of the rheumatoid forefoot
- the material characteristics and the presence of seams also warrant extra consideration where there is a risk of ulceration secondary to impaired arterial supply or vasculitis
- increased pressure found under the rheumatoid forefoot is aided by the addition of cushioning, provided separately or incorporated into prescription footwear
- rigid/semi-rigid, functional orthoses are known to be effective in limiting the rate of hindfoot and forefoot deformity, and in redistributing load away from the forefoot

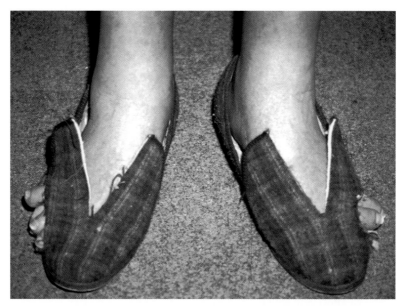

Figure 8.4 Self-help by a patient with RA who requires non-standard footwear.

- standard laces can be changed for elastic laces in existing shoes, removing the need for the wearer to bend and tie them
- alternative fastenings such as Velcro or elastic should be considered when choosing or prescribing orthopaedic footwear.

Juvenile idiopathic arthritis

Definition

Juvenile idiopathic arthritis (JIA) is a heterogeneous group of inflammatory arthropathies indicated by the presence of an inflammatory arthropathy with an onset at less than 16 years of age, affecting one or more joints for longer than 6 weeks.

Epidemiology

Around 12 000 children in the UK have JIA and girls are almost three times more likely to be affected than boys. Classification systems can be found in the main book.

For more information see
Neale's Disorders of the Foot 8E   *pages 211–212*

Diagnosis

This is based on the exclusion of other provisional diagnoses such as infection and trauma.

History is usually of a chronic idiopathic synovitis, onset being in a single joint, typically the knee, ankle, hip or wrist (oligoarticular onset).

Blood tests are less helpful than in adult-onset arthritis, but can help the clinician to decide to which sub-group the patient belongs.

Pathophysiology is specific to the sub-group, but is essentially that of a chronic immune-mediated inflammatory synovitis.

Onset is often before 4 years of age and the clinical course is variable and dependent on the clinical sub-group.

Medical management

- General principle is of support rather than cure, and is aimed at limiting symptoms, maintaining function and minimising permanent changes
- Non-steroidal anti-inflammatory drugs (NSAIDs) will be the initial intervention
- Intra-articular steroids are often used.

Particular attention should be given to the feet in JIA as deformity will occur quickly.

In-shoe orthoses must be reviewed annually, and more frequently during growth spurts.

Seronegative inflammatory arthritis

Introduction – common features

- Known association with the human leukocyte antigen (HLA) B27
- Clinically frequent involvement of the spine (axial involvement)
- Inflammatory process associated with enthesopathy
- Most common sites for enthesopathy in the foot are the posterior calcaneus at the insertion of the tendo Achilles, the plantar calcaneus (the plantar fascia, and the short flexor muscles), the base of the fifth metatarsal and the forefoot
- In the toes the enthesitis and synovitis can present with marked dactylitis or 'sausage digits' Fig 8.5

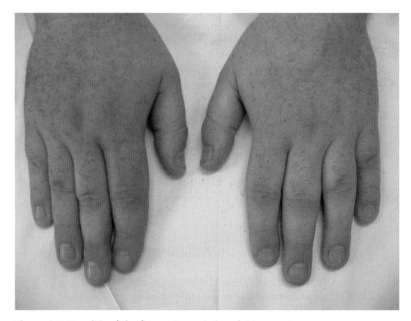

Figure 8.5 Dactylitis of the fingers in psoriatic arthritis.

- More widespread inflammation can lead to noticeable general swelling in the foot.

Ankylosing spondylitis

- A progressive seronegative spondyloarthropathy that affects the axial skeleton (the spine and surrounding structures) predominantly, but which also has peripheral features that can involve the foot
- Incidence of ankylosing spondylitis (AS) is approximately 1%, with men affected by AS three times as frequently as women
- Diagnosis is based on the modified New York criteria of one of the following:
  - inflammatory back pain >3 months' duration
  - limited spinal mobility in two planes
  - limited chest expansion, plus evidence of sacroiliitis on plain X-ray
- Pathology is not well understood overall, but appears driven by enthesitis
- The sacroiliac joints are the worst affected
- NSAIDs are the mainstay of medical management in AS
- About 20% of patients with AS will have enthesitis in the feet
- Erosions, periosteal proliferation and, characteristically, joint ankylosis are all seen
- Joints appear swollen and tender
- Radiographic investigation reveals that initial periarticular erosion is followed by bony proliferation, and bone spur formation
- Management of AS in the foot centres on systemic disease control supplemented with local measures
- Where isolated sites in the foot are symptomatic, local injection of corticosteroid may reduce inflammation and padding or orthoses may provide mechanical relief.

Psoriatic arthritis

- An inflammatory arthropathy occurring in the presence of psoriasis and in the absence of rheumatoid factor
- Spinal involvement is characteristic, but peripheral joint involvement may range from the widespread and severe arthritis seen in the form *arthritis mutilans* to a relatively mild monoarthritis
- Psoriasis of the skin or nails affects between 2 and 3% of the population, with approximately 12% of dermatologic cases developing arthritis
- No widely agreed diagnostic criteria for psoriatic arthritis
- Diagnosis is based on clinical features and the often difficult exclusion of other inflammatory arthritides such as RA and ankylosing spondylitis
- Medical management for psoriatic arthritis is often similar to that of RA, with methotrexate and other DMARDs proving effective in combination with NSAIDs and exercise
- Foot may show the changes typical of psoriatic skin disease:
  - erythematous patches on the extensor surfaces or plantar hyperkeratosis or pustule formation on the plantar surfaces
  - pitting, discoloration, hyperkeratosis and lysis of the nails and splinter haemorrhages may be found around the apices of toes
  - psoriatic arthritis will often present initially in the interphalangeal and then the MP joints of the feet or hands, although other joints may be affected, sometimes in a single ray pattern
  - inflammation at the entheses results in bony erosions

- radiographic investigations show non-marginal erosions early, with subchondral bone involved soon afterwards
- reactive new bone formation around affected joints is characteristic, leading to a fuzzy appearance on X-ray
- endosteal sclerosis will occasionally lead to a substantial increase in density of the shaft, the so-called 'ivory phalanx'
- the highly erosive pathology leads to a whittling of the joint margins and an unusual 'pencil in cup' appearance in advanced cases where the distal end of the affected phalanx is cupped within an excessively concave surface at the proximal end of the more distal phalanx
- conversely, bony ankylosis can occur instead
- resorption of the distal phalanx occurs resulting in a characteristic, pointed toe pulp
- hindfoot involvement mimics that of other seronegative arthropathies
- clinical involvement of the tendo Achilles and plantar fasciitis occurs.

Reactive arthritis

- Can occur in conjunction with urethritis and conjunctivitis
- An acute inflammatory arthritis arising after a local or systemic infection, typically sexually acquired or post-dysenteric
- Disease usually affects younger males and is associated with the HLA B27 antigen
- Initial presentation usually in the knee or foot
- Spondyloarthropathy is a universal feature as the disease progresses
- Disease course is of flares and remissions which will self limit in time
- A small proportion of cases will persist but the disease tends to be milder than other inflammatory arthropathies
- Reactive arthritis should be suspected where there is an inflammatory arthritis presenting predominantly in the lower limb, especially where the arthritis is accompanied by bony proliferation
- Multiple joints may be affected but usually asymmetrically
- Most commonly affected regions in the foot are the MP joints, the tendo Achilles and its insertion, and the origin of the plantar fascia
- NSAIDs are the first-line treatment, reducing pain and subduing the inflammatory process to some degree
- Often a course of DMARDs is all that is necessary.

The foot

- Involvement in the foot largely mirrors that of other seronegative arthropathies, focussing on the hindfoot and, to a lesser extent, the forefoot, but largely sparing the midfoot
- Whiskery spurs resulting from enthesopathy at the insertion of the tendo Achilles and plantar fascia
- Nodular thickenings may also be found in the tendons.

Connective tissue diseases – scleroderma and lupus

Connective tissue diseases (CTDs) are a mixed group of conditions sharing some clinical features, but with differing pathophysiology.

The two most common discrete forms are scleroderma and systemic lupus erythematosus (commonly known as lupus).

Scleroderma

This comes in several forms including progressive systemic sclerosis and localised or limited sclerosis. It is an immune-mediated disorder characterised by inflammatory and fibrotic soft-tissue changes. In the systemic form, vascular lesions are also characteristic, affecting the skin and internal structures, such as gastrointestinal system, heart, lungs and kidneys.

The gender split is 1 : 4 male : female.

Anti-nuclear antibodies are usually present in the blood, and extractable nuclear antibodies to SCL-70, centromere and RNP may be found; as may rheumatoid factor.

Pathology

The precise pathology is unknown:

- initial presentation of systemic sclerosis may simply be with Raynaud's phenomenon accompanied by oedema of the hands or feet.
- the skin in the extremities thickens and tightens leading to the typical presentation of sclerodactyly.
- the affected fingers and toes develop flexion contractures that cause limited mobility. Fig 8.6
- fibrosis and resorption of the soft-tissue and underlying bony substance of the digital apices can lead to a classical atrophic appearance to the ends of the digits.
- changes in the face lead to a mask-like appearance, with puckering of the skin around the mouth.
- altered pigmentation is common.
- one variant of scleroderma is the CREST syndrome, named after the features Calcinosis, Raynaud's phenomenon, oEsophagitis, Sclerodactyly and Telangectiasis.
- in CREST the scleroderma is usually limited to the hands and forearms.

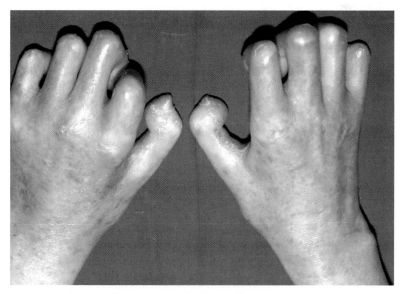

Figure 8.6 Fibrosis and contracture in the hands of a patient with scleroderma.

- calcinosis manifests as small subcutaneous nodules on the hands and feet resembling gouty tophi clinically, but clearly showing themselves as containing calcium on plain X-rays.
- CREST is not a benign condition.
- there is a high prevalence of lung and heart involvement.
- systemic scleroderma pulmonary, cardiac and renal involvement leads to shortening of the lifespan.
- synovitis may be present, but tends to affect large joints rather than the feet.
- calcification of peripheral soft tissues may occur in long-standing cases and calcinosis of the skin may be seen.

The foot

- Localised vasculitic lesions and ulceration, typically of the dorsum of the forefoot and apices of toes
- Raynaud's syndrome
- Subcutaneous calcinosis can be problematic
- Ulcerative skin lesions are often very painful in CTD patients
- Healing is typically protracted because of the vasculitis, and when healing does occur it is often through necrosis and fibrosis
- Combination of skin and subcutaneous fibrosis, along with the changes in the underlying skeletal structures lead to difficulties with shoe fitting.

Lupus

- Systemic lupus erythematosus (SLE) – an immune-mediated connective tissue disease affecting many organ systems and with a variable course and prognosis
- In addition to the musculoskeletal effects, renal and cardiopulmonary diseases are common features
- Discoid lupus is a localised form affecting only the skin
- SLE is between 2 and 8x more common in women than in men
- Characteristic malar 'butterfly rash' on the cheeks
- Diagnosis made on the basis of an 11-item set of criteria, including physical characteristics and laboratory investigations such as HLA typing, detection of antinuclear antibodies and antibodies to double-stranded DNA
- NSAID therapy is used sparingly because of an increased risk of renal dysfunction
- Anti-malarials are effective for mild SLE
- Mainstays of therapy are steroids and immunosuppressive drugs.

The foot

- Vascular signs occur
- Telangectasia and purpura affecting the feet widely
- Vasculitis and ulceration are relatively common
- In addition to the small vessel vasculitis seen in RA, people with lupus can also develop large vessel vasculitis and accelerated atherosclerosis leading to frank gangrene and risk of amputation
- Ankle-brachial pressure indices are abnormal in many lupus sufferers and should be used to detect large vessel disease early in this group
- Patients with SLE may have RA-type presentations in the feet
- Tendinopathy can be seen, especially in the tendo Achilles
- Patients can present with onycholysis and pitting of the nails, similar to that seen in psoriasis

- Splinter haemorrhages in the nail beds reflect the vascular involvement
- Skin lesions are common, with discoid or annular erythematous lesions occurring on the legs and feet exacerbated by exposure to sunlight.

Osteoarthritis

There is progressive loss of articular cartilage, and remodelling and change in the structure of subchondral bone:

- most common sites are the hands (1%), hips (0.9%), knees (2.4%) and feet
- clinical signs – general stiffness and an aching pain in the affected joint
- there may be tenderness at the joint margins on palpation
- crepitus may be felt on passive movement of the part
- confirmation of the clinical signs requires radiographic investigation
- radiographic signs featured in the Menz system include narrowing of the joint space on plain X-ray, bony proliferation around joint margins (osteophyte formation) and sclerosis and cyst formation in the subchondral bone
- periarticular erosions are not seen in osteoarthritis (OA).

This is no longer considered simple 'wear and tear' arthritis, as it is clear that the process involves elements of repair as well as inflammation and degeneration.

The risk factors for OA include inherent factors such as age, ethnicity and gender, combined with acquired factors such as local mechanics, obesity, trauma and deformity.

Primary osteoarthritis is a significant inflammatory element:

- significant pain, especially early on in the disease process
- osteophytes develop at the margins of the articular surfaces near the attachments of the capsule, ligaments or tendons
- endochondral ossification follows, spreading to involve neighbouring soft-tissue structures. In both primary and secondary presentations the cartilage reduces in thickness as the matrix degenerates, especially in regions of higher stresses
- chondrocyte biochemistry leads to a self-promoting degenerative cascade hastening the process of deterioration
- the subchondral bone becomes sclerotic and cysts become evident, again in areas of high stress
- the soft-tissue structures, such as the synovium and ligaments, can be involved but not to the extent seen in the inflammatory arthritides.

Medical management

This still relies on the traditional pyramid approach:

- education and self-management are central features of the national standards of care for OA
- the first MTPJ is a highly prevalent site for joint degeneration, second only to the knee
- other joints in the foot are affected more sporadically, most often following trauma
- proximal foot joints in the tarsus and tarsometatarsal region showed degeneration
- most common presentation of OA in the foot is as hallux limitus, hallux rigidus or in association with hallux valgus
- degenerative changes at the 1st MTPJ lead to functional limitation

- pain and stiffness are felt in the affected joint, especially in maximal dorsiflexion, and this may interfere with normal walking
- periarticular osteophyte formation leads to thickening of the 1st MTPJ, and sometimes the formation of an adventitious bursa
- the osteophytic change will be evident on plain X-ray, as will joint space narrowing
- the limitation of joint range of movement may be progressive, with decreasing range associated with increasing impairment
- weight loss and low-impact exercise are of known benefit and some effort should be directed towards exercise counselling during the clinical consultation
- contoured foot orthoses, provided either to a neutral cast or off the shelf, are effective at reducing foot joint motions and offloading the forefoot and heel regions, and so may help some patients
- similarly, shock-absorbing insoles or footwear can provide symptom relief and accommodative padding may reduce pressure over prominences resulting from osteoarthritic changes
- footwear adaptations such as rocker-bottom shoes limit the need for movement of degenerate joints while facilitating sagittal plane motion
- intra-articular injection of steroid may provide symptom relief for up to 8 weeks
- surgical intervention is usually definitive with arthrodesis, or replacement or excision arthroplasty reducing pain significantly.

Crystal arthropathies (gout and pseudo gout)

- Clinical manifestations of an inflammatory response to crystal deposition in STJs
- Gout occurs in around 1% of men and 0.3–0.6% of women and the incidence increases with age, being rare in adults under 30 years of age
- Pseudogout is much less common and is predominantly a disease of the elderly
- Crystals may be viewed directly within joint aspirate under polarised light microscopy
- The clinical picture in true gout is usually obvious
- Microscopy is often only confirmatory, although joint aspiration should always be performed to exclude septic arthritis or coincidental degenerative or inflammatory arthritis
- Underlying pathology of gout is of crystal deposition into the joint space as a result of elevated levels of monosodium urate in the blood stream
- Pseudogout occurs when calcium pyrophosphate dihydrate, a normal component of articular cartilage, enters the joint space and is taken up by white cells
- A less common form is caused by deposition of calcium hydroxapatite
- The local pathology within the affected joint is of crystal deposition leading to severe synovitis
- Synovial proliferation occurs and the inflammatory cascade is instigated and modulated by leucocytes, monocytes and lymphocytes
- Tophi are the consequence of phagocytosis of crystals, and are composed of high concentrations of crystals and the detritus of deceased polymorphs.

Four phases of gout include:

1. asymptomatic hyperuricaemia
2. acute gouty arthritis

3. intercritical gout
4. chronic tophaceous gout.

Initial presentation is typically a severe and acute monoarthritis lasting a few days.

Preceding an acute attack there may be a history of precipitating factors, such as dietary change, an alcohol binge or minor trauma to the joint.

Onset is rapid/overnight with a rapid development of a severe monoarthritis manifest as heat, redness and marked swelling.

More diffuse swelling can result if more than one joint is involved:

- medical management of the acute phase for all crystal arthropathies is with high therapeutic doses of NSAID.
- other therapies such as oral steroid are available for patients unable to tolerate high doses of NSAIDs but are not preferred.
- colchicine is only appropriate in the earliest stages of an acute episode of gout.
- oral or injected steroid may be of assistance where single or few accessible joints are involved.
- local therapies such as the application of ice may be helpful.
- preventative regimens of drugs such as low-dose colchicine, uric clearance promoters such as Probenecid, and the xanthine oxidase inhibitor Allopurinol can be effective in reducing the frequency of subsequent attacks when combined with dietary modification.

For some time now patients who were allergic to allopurinol had no alternatives. Now there is an inhibitor of xanthine oxidase – Febuxostat. Febuxostat is as good or better than Allopurinol in reducing the concentration of uric acid in the blood and has now been approved by NICE for those people who cannot take Allopurinol.

The foot in crystal arthropathies

- True gout will onset in the 1st MTPJ in about half of all cases.
- It also has a predilection for other sites in the foot such as the other MTPJs, the 1st interphalangeal (IP) joint, midfoot joints, the STJ and the ankle.
- Pseudogout presents with a less severe synovitis and affects larger joints such as the ankle and knee.
- Crystal arthropathies are characterised by a hyper acute monoarthritis, accompanied by severe swelling erythema and pain.
- The joint will typically be too painful to move or to touch.

Infective arthritis

Infective (septic) arthritis is a direct response to the presence of infective organisms (usually bacteria) in the joint and so usually presents as an acute monoarthritis, often with an accompanying systemic presentation of fever. It is uncommon in the foot joints, preferring larger joints such as the knee.

Infective arthritis is more common in children than adults.

The foot in infective arthritis

- Although the foot is rarely affected, infective arthritis can occur secondary to ulceration or following a penetrating injury.
- It is more prevalent in people with sensory neuropathy.
- It should be considered in the case of an acute monoarthritis in the foot after surgery.

- It requires aspiration of joint fluids and long-term antibiotic therapy, but will usually resolve completely.

OTHER RHEUMATOLOGICAL CONDITIONS

Fibromyalgia

- Fibromyalgia (FM) is a label given to a presentation of chronic, widespread pain in both muscles and joints.
- Diagnosis is on the basis of 11 or more tender points at specific sites in the body.
- Prevalence is estimated at 1–2%, the majority of cases arising in females.
- It is associated with higher scores on anxiety and depression scales.
- Prevalence increases with age.
- Patients report chronic musculoskeletal fatigue and pain, often severe enough to interfere with ability to work and participate in leisure activities.
- The clinical course is variable, but fairly poor.

Medical management

- Management is directed towards management of chronic pain and its attendant psychological effects.
- Pain relief is required, usually using analgesics or NSAIDs, although these may not be effective alone.
- Managing the psychological aspects of FM may be helpful.
- Selective serotonin reuptake inhibitors (SSRIs) or tricyclic antidepressants such as amitriptyline are often prescribed.
- Antidepressants may be combined with non-pharmaceutical approaches such as exercise and cognitive behavioural therapy.
- Exercise has been demonstrated to improve outcomes in patients with fibromyalgia.
- The foot is not an especially common site for involvement.

Polymyalgia rheumatica

- A musculoskeletal pain syndrome usually seen in females over 65 years
- Affects about seven people per thousand
- Musculoskeletal symptoms occur mainly around the upper (in the shoulders and neck) and lower (buttocks and upper thighs) limb girdles
- Onset of symptoms may be dramatic over a few days and can lead to severe disability. Systemic symptoms such as fever and night sweats may occur, as may weight loss
- Pathology is unknown
- Clinical course is of diffuse musculoskeletal pain early and because of its dramatic course patients usually present early
- Treatment with NSAIDs may help but low-dose oral steroids have an equally dramatic benefit on the symptoms, this response being part of the criteria for diagnosis
- Polymyalgia rheumatica does not affect the feet directly, but patients with difficulty bending and with reduced grip strength due to the disease may need assistance with basic foot care.

Sjögren's syndrome

- A CTD affecting the salivary and tear glands
- Relatively rare and may occur as a primary forms, i.e. in the absence of any other disease, or in a secondary form associated with other rheumatic diseases such as RA or lupus
- Main effects are dryness of the mucous membranes, especially the eyes and mouth. The skin can be affected also, and anhydrosis is the most common manifestation in the foot. Patients can benefit from education about the importance of an emollient regimen, including footbaths and creams
- Sjögren's syndrome can be associated with vasculitis, and the toes can be involved
- Management is the same as for the other forms of vasculitis in the rheumatology clinic.

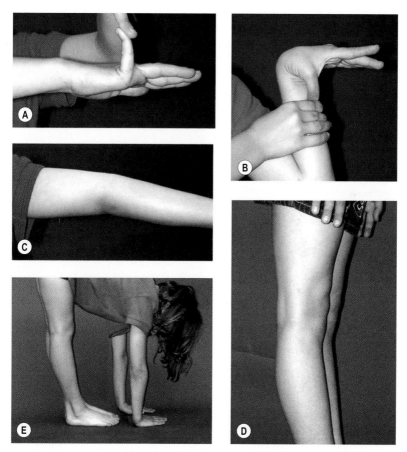

Figure 8.7 The Beighton-Carter-Wilkinson scale for assessing joint hypermobility (A) Hyperextension of the fingers past 90°. (B) Touch the thumb to the volar aspect of forearm. (C) Elbow hyperextension >10°. (D) Knee hyperextension >10°. (E) Being able to place palms flat on the floor with knees extended. One point is given to each positive sign (one point for each positive limb for signs A–D) to yield a score out of 9.

Joint hypermobility syndromes

- Several conditions are associated with a generalised hypermobility of joints
- The most common are the benign familial joint hypermobility syndrome, the nine basic classifications of Ehlers–Danlos disease, Marfan syndrome and osteogenesis imperfecta
- Diagnosis of hypermobility made on the basis of the well-known Beighton score a five-item, nine-point scale recording the physical features associated with systemic joint laxity Fig 8.7
- Pathology of hypermobility syndrome derives from disordered structure of Types I and III collagen
- Gradation in bundle size is lost, and Type I : Type III ratios are deranged leading to decreased tensile strength of connective tissues in the skin and articular structures
- Tendency to easy bruising and papyraceous scars from impaired healing
- Multiple intermittent joint and soft-tissue pain, with pain in the back, hands, wrists and shoulders being at least as common as lower-limb problems
- Develop similar sorts of 'overuse' type symptoms as the rest of the population (tenosynovitis, arthralgia and so on) but do so more frequently and more severe
- Treatment aimed at symptom relief
- Mainstays are NSAIDs and selective local corticosteroid in the short term, combined with physical and occupational therapy
- Exercises to strengthen and stabilise affected joints
- Rehabilitation strategies including proprioception training.

Chapter | 9 |

Metabolic disorders

Metabolic disorders are important with regard to public health and may result in significant disease to the foot. They include diabetes, obesity and metabolic bone disorders.

DIABETES MELLITUS

Is a persistently raised blood glucose level due to:
- reduced production of insulin
- impaired effectiveness of insulin.

Diabetes mellitus can be divided into:
- type 1 (previously IDDM)
- type 2 (previously NIDDM)
- secondary diabetes.

Type 1 diabetes mellitus

- A complete lack of effective insulin
- Usually occurs in children and before 30 years of age
- May present in middle age and in the elderly.

Type 2 diabetes mellitus

- A relative lack of insulin
- Peripheral tissue becomes insulin-resistant
- Usually presents after 40 years of age
- Obesity is not unusual.

Secondary diabetes

Occurs due to direct damage, removal or impairment of action of beta cells. It is uncommon, but causes include:

- severe malnutrition
- pancreatic destruction
- haemochromatosis
- pancreatectomy
- antagonism to action of insulin
- drugs
- pregnancy (gestational diabetes).

Diagnosis

The standard oral glucose tolerance test is rarely required:

- a random blood glucose of more than 11.1 mmol/l
- fasting blood glucose of a 75 g glucose load is greater than 7.0 mmol/l and greater than 11.1 mmol/l at 2 hours.

Clinical features

The classic symptoms are:

- thirst
- polyuria and nocturia
- weight loss
- pruritus vulvae or balanitis
- more severe symptoms or more acute in type 1 diabetes.

The symptoms of type 1 diabetes occur over a few weeks and lead to:

- muscle wasting
- physical weakness
- vomiting and dehydration
- urgent need for insulin
- ketoacidosis, which presents as:
  - drowsiness
  - dehydration
  - over-breathing (together with acetone in the breath).

In cases of ketoacidosis urgent admission to hospital and insulin therapy is required.

Treatment

Treatment of type 1 diabetes

- Insulin replacement therapy:
  - human insulin is used by the majority of patients
  - insulin analogues are also available
- Diet – regular carbohydrate intake at fixed times
- Exercise
- During infection or illness blood glucose increases insulin dose is increased.

Treatment of type 2 diabetes

Treatment requires lowering of insulin requirements. Three measures are available for treatment:

- diet – 50% of the calorie intake should be carbohydrates and no more than 35% fats
- exercise
- hypoglycaemic agents:
  - sulphonylureas
  - biguanides

- acarbose
- thioglitazones.

Insulin is sometimes required.

Hypoglycaemia

Symptoms of hypoglycaemia usually occur when the blood glucose is less than 3 mmol/l.

Symptoms fall into two groups.

- Sympathetic symptoms:
  - shaking
  - trembling
  - sweating
  - pins and needles in the tongue and lips
- Neuroglycopaenic mild symptoms:
  - double vision
  - difficulty in concentrating
  - slurring of speech
  - moderate symptoms are:
    - confusion
    - change in behaviour
    - truculence
  - late symptoms are:
    - epileptic fits especially in children
    - hemiplegia in the elderly
    - unconsciousness.

Treatment

If the patient is conscious:

- oral glucose as a drink
- tablet or gel
- followed by biscuits or sandwiches.

The unconscious patient should be:

- placed in the recovery position, airway maintained
- treated with intravenous (iv) glucose
- given a further dose of iv glucose after 5 minutes if no response
- given intramuscular glucagon.

Complications and control of diabetes

Diabetic patients may develop a variety of complications:

- microvascular disease (retinopathy and nephropathy)
- nervous system abnormalities
- macrovascular disease (coronary, peripheral vascular and cerebral vascular disease).

Eye disease

Diabetes is the most common cause of blindness under the age of 65 in the UK.

Kidney disease

Type 1 diabetes is responsible for the majority of cases in those under 50 years of age.

Neuropathy

Table 9.1 Classification of diabetic neuropathies

Progressive	Symmetrical sensory polyneuropathy and autonomic neuropathy
Reversible	Acute painful neuropathies, radiculopathies and mononeuropathies (including proximal motor neuropathy/ femoral neuropathy and diabetic amyotrophy)
Pressure palsies	Carpal tunnel syndrome Ulnar nerve depression Foot drops

Table 9.2 Leg abnormalities in diabetes

	NEUROPATHY	**ISCHAEMIA**
Symptoms	None Paraesthesia Pain Oedema Painful wasted thigh Foot drop	None Claudication Rest pain
Structural damage	Ulcer Sepsis Abscess Osteomyelitis Digital gangrene Charcot joints	Ulcer Sepsis Gangrene

Vascular disease

- Atheromatous arterial disease with a peripheral distribution in the legs
- Medial arterial calcification (Monckeberg's sclerosis) of distal arteries
- Symptomless myocardial infarction is more common in diabetes.

The diabetic foot

The foot in diabetes can be affected by:
- neuropathies. Table 9.1
- circulatory changes
- trauma and infection.

The diabetic foot can be divided into:

- the neuropathic foot: Table 9.2
  - warm, numb, dry and usually painless foot
  - palpable pulses

- three complications:
  - the neuropathic ulcer
  - neuropathic (Charcot) foot
  - rarely neuropathic oedema
- the neuroischaemic foot:
  - cool foot
  - absent pedal pulses
  - three complications:
    - rest pain
    - ulceration
    - gangrene
- the ischaemic foot with no concomitant neuropathy is rarely seen.

The neuropathic foot

Neuropathic ulcer

Patient unaware of ulceration due to loss of pain sensation. Direct mechanical injuries to the plantar surface result from treading on nails and sharp objects. The most frequent cause of ulceration is neglect of high-pressure areas with overlying callous.

Complications

- Infection
- Impaired inflammatory response
- Cellulitis
- Tracking of infection involving underlying tendons, bones and joints
- Necrotising infection
- Gangrene.

Management

- Removal of excess callous
- Expose base of ulcer
- Allow efficient drainage
- Bacteriological swab from base of the ulcer
- Prescribe appropriate oral antibiotics until the ulcer has healed:
  - amoxicillin, 500 mg t.d.s., for streptococcal infections
  - flucloxacillin, 500 mg q.d.s., for staphylococcal infections
  - metronidazole, 400 mg t.d.s., for anaerobic infections
  - ciprofloxacin, 500 mg b.d. for Gram-negative infections
  - superficial ulcers with no cellulitis are treated as inpatients
  - presence of cellulitis or skin discoloration requires urgent hospitalisation
- Re-distribution of weight-bearing forces with:
  - special footwear
  - moulded insoles
  - total-contact cast
  - Scotchcast boot
  - Aircast (walking brace).

Neuropathic (Charcot's) joint

The metatarsal–tarsal joints are most commonly involved. Caused by trauma to an area which results in unilateral:

- swelling
- erythema

- heat
- pain.

Serial radiographs show evidence of:

- bony fracture
- osteolysis
- fragmentation
- new bone formation
- subluxation and joint disorganisation.

Management

- Immobilisation of the injured area
- Non-weight bearing with crutches or a total contact plaster cast
- Gradual mobilisation using a moulded insole and special footwear.

Neuropathic oedema

Swelling of the feet and lower legs associated with severe peripheral neuropathy is very uncommon. Ephedrine, 30 mg t.d.s is a useful treatment.

The neuroischaemic foot

Pathogenesis

In diabetic patients atherosclerosis is multisegmental, bilateral and distal involving the popliteal, tibial and peroneal arteries.

Clinical features

- Intermittent claudication
- Rest pain
- Ulceration:
  - surrounded by a rim of erythema
  - callous absent
  - painful (unless peripheral neuropathy co-exists)
- Gangrene
- Sites of ulceration are:
  - tips of toes
  - medial surface of 1st metatarsal head
  - lateral surface of 5th metatarsal head
  - heel.

Management

Medical management for small, shallow ulcers of recent onset includes the following:

- painful ulcers – prescribe opiates
- removal of necrotic tissue from ulcers
- bacteriology swabs from floor of ulcer
- ulcers cleansed
- non-adherent sterile dressings
- specific antibiotic therapy.

Surgical management is required for severe sepsis:

- emergency hospitalisation
- control of sepsis by intravenous antibiotics
- surgical debridement

- revascularisation by angioplasty or reconstruction if appropriate
- footwear to accommodate the foot.

OBESITY

The most common assessment is through the measurement of weight in relation to height and age. The body mass index (bmi) is commonly used and equals weight (in kg) over height (in metres); the normal range is up to 25.

Aetiology

- Genetic
- Environmental
- Socio-economic factors
- Endocrine diseases, hypothyroidism and Cushing's syndrome are rarely a cause of obesity.

Major long-term health hazards are:

- hypertension
- coronary artery disease
- breathlessness
- backache
- increased risk of morbidity and mortality.

Treatment

- Exclude myxoedema and Cushing's syndrome
- Reduce calorie intake
- Patient in control of weight reduction
- Medical treatments to decrease appetite have a limited role
- Prolonged behavioural courses
- Surgical treatments:
  - intestinal bypass
  - gastric stapling
  - gastric balloons
  - wiring of the jaws
  - surgical removal of excess adipose tissue.

METABOLIC BONE DISEASE

This involves the bone and calcium metabolism.

Hypercalcaemia

The commonest causes of hypercalcaemia are:

- malignancy
- hyperparathyroidism.

  Any tendency to hypercalcaemia can be aggravated by:

- dehydration
- impaired renal function
- immobilisation or fracture.

Clinical signs

- Patients feel generally ill
- Patients feel depressed
- May be misdiagnosed with a psychological disorder
- Severe hypercalcaemia produces:
  - confusion
  - coma
  - anuria
  - death through cardiac arrest.

Treatment

- Identify cause
- Rehydration
- Diuresis encouraged by intravenous fluid infusion and loop diuretics
- Steroids can be effective, especially in malignancy.

Hypocalcaemia

In hypocalcaemia and tetany there may be:

- peripheral paraesthesia
- muscle cramps
- epileptic fits
- laryngeal spasm in children
- acute hypertension
- psychosis
- important physical signs, Chvostek's and Trousseau's.

Treatment

- In emergencies slow intravenous injection of calcium gluconate
- In the long term, dietary calcium is supplemented and a vitamin D preparation administered.

Osteoporosis

This is the loss of the structural integrity of the internal architecture of bone. Less bone is present than normal for the patient's age and sex.

Two forms encountered frequently are the senile and related postmenopausal osteoporosis.

Common sites include:

- spine
- proximal femur
- foot and ankle
- toe and metatarsal fractures.

Diagnosis

Exclude:

- osteomalacia
- renal pathology
- hyperparathyroidism.

Treatment

Reduce the rate of bone loss by:

- adequate calcium intake
- female hormone replacement therapy
- regular physical exercise
- diet with a daily intake of 1–1.5 g calcium per day
- severe cases: drug therapy including bisphosphonates, raloxifene and parathyroid hormone.

Osteomalacia and rickets

Osteomalacia and rickets occur when there is defective mineralisation of the bone matrix. In rickets the defect is present in infancy and childhood.

Osteomalacia

This is the adult counterpart of rickets.

Aetiology

Three main groups:

- Nutritional
- Malabsorptive
- Renal.

Clinical signs and symptoms

- Bone and muscle tenderness
- Aching pain adjacent to an affected portion of the tibia
- Increased warmth in the anterior leg
- Bony deformity results from weight bearing
- Degenerative arthritis of both the ankle and knee joints.

Rickets

This is not seen until after the patient is 1 year old.

Clinical signs and symptoms

- Swelling of the ankles and wrists
- Tiredness
- Muscular weakness
- Bone pain
- Pain on movement
- Delayed dentition and deformed teeth
- Swelling and tenderness of distal ends of the radius and ulna
- Rickety rosary (costochondral swellings)
- Frontal and parietal bossing of the skull occurs
- Bowing of the legs may result from weight bearing
- Kyphoscoliosis
- Radiographs show:
  - widening and decreased density of the line of calcification
  - irregularity and concavity of the metaphysis
  - rarefaction with deformities in the bone shaft.

Treatment

- Rickets and osteomalacia:
  - vitamin D or one of its potent derivatives – alfacalcidol or calcitriol
  - long-term maintenance dosage of one of the derivatives
  - surgical correction of deformity is occasionally required.

Hyperparathyroidism

Hyperparathyroidism presents as a form of osteoporosis with a fracture. Occasionally the giant cell tumour associated with severe hyperparathyroidism may present as a mass in the tibia.

Renal osteodystrophy

The main bone changes that occur are:

- osteomalacia
- secondary hypoparathyroidism
- steroid-treated renal patients present vascular necrosis of the talus associated with renal transplant.

Management

- Treatment with phosphate-binding agents or a low-phosphate diet
- Vitamin D therapy in hypoparathyroidism and vitamin D deficiency osteomalacia
- Parathyroidectomy in severe secondary hyperparathyroidism.

Paget's disease

Paget's disease is a focal disorder of bone remodelling characterised by excessive osteoclastic resorption. Usually occurs over the age of 40 years.

Clinical features

- Bone pain
- Degenerative joint disease
- Neurological symptoms from involvement of the spine, leading to paraplegia
- Neuropathies of the cranial and peripheral nerves may occur secondary to entrapment
- Radiological abnormality is resorption of a previously normal cortex.

Treatment

- Drug therapy to inhibit bone resorption.

Chapter 10

Management of high-risk patients

The main aims when managing high-risk patients, be they diabetic or not, are summarised below:

- to prevent complications (for example, infection or injury)
- to effectively manage established wounds, infection or necrosis.

PREVENTION OF COMPLICATIONS

History taking and assessment

Obtaining a detailed medical history is paramount; this is accompanied by a vascular, neurological and biomechanical assessment – see the various chapters in this textbook.

For more information see
Neale's Disorders of the Foot 8E   *pages 244–245*

General points regarding treatment

The practitioner must pay close attention to aseptic/antiseptic techniques. The use of autoclaves for instrument sterilisation is mandatory. Meticulous pre-operative preparation of the patient's skin is necessary to effect a rapid reduction in the number of pathogenic transient flora, and to remove gross contamination. The most important pre-operative cleansing routine is a thorough application of an alcohol-based preparation; any antiseptic that is added to the alcohol provides limited improvement to the solution's activity.

Padding must be accurately shaped, avoiding creases and irregularities. Strapping should be non-constrictive. If caustic medicaments are used they must be applied with great care and their actions monitored closely. Detailed advice regarding suitable footwear and hosiery is essential and is considered in other chapters. Minor surgical procedures are performed as a last resort, and only after consultation with the patient's general practitioner.

Box 10.1 **History of the wound**

1. The DURATION of the wound
2. Any changes in the SIZE or APPEARANCE of the wound?
3. Any change in the NUMBER of lesions/wounds?
4. Any PREVIOUS INCIDENTS of similar lesions?
5. Any PAIN or ALTERED SENSATION associated with the lesion?
6. The presence of other SIGNS and/or SYMPTOMS that may be related to the wound, e.g. ischaemic changes
7. Does the patient know the CAUSE of the wound?

MANAGEMENT OF ESTABLISHED WOUNDS, INFECTION OR NECROSIS

An ulcer is an example of a wound that, for various reasons, will not heal. Most research pertinent to wound healing is not restricted to ulcers; the general term 'wound' is used in preference to the term 'ulcer' in the following discussion.

The following wound-management strategies are considered:

- examination of the wound
- the use of antiseptics and topical medicaments
- the use of dressings.

Examination of the wound

A detailed history and examination of the wound should take place at the initial consultation (Box 10.1).

At each subsequent visit the wound and the patient's general condition are assessed, any changes being recorded with meticulous care. The points that will be observed by the podiatrist are summarised in Box 10.2 and Figure 10.1.

Photographs provide a detailed permanent record and pieces of sterile transparent film, often as part of wound-dressing systems, are available.

Management of wounds

- The most effective method of preventing contamination is to reduce conversation while attending to the wound and to carry out well-organised treatment.
- Sterile surgical gloves may be worn, particularly when working on deep wounds, but clean latex gloves are acceptable, providing that they are replaced frequently, and worn only at appropriate times.
- Three levels of hand-washing are recognised: social hand-washing (using soap and water), hygienic hand-washing (with antiseptic hand-wash preparation), and, finally, surgical hand-washing (a 3-minute hand-wash using an antiseptic). At all levels washing must be performed so that all surfaces of the hands are treated.
- Single-use plastic aprons may be worn to prevent contamination of permeable cotton clinic coats.
- The use of pre-packed, sterile instruments, medicaments and dressings is part of normal practice, and aseptic techniques should be employed correctly and with care.

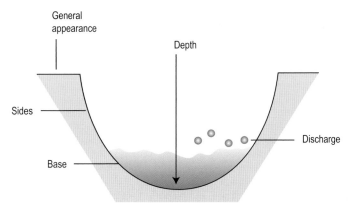

Figure 10.1 Points to observe when examining a wound.

Box 10.2 Points to observe when examining a wound

1. The precise ANATOMICAL SITE of the wound
2. The SIZE of the wound. This should be measured accurately using a commercial measuring device
3. The GENERAL APPEARANCE of the wound and the surrounding tissue, e.g. presence of callus or maceration. Special note should be made of signs of local or spreading infection (cellulitis, lymphangitis, lymphadenitis)
4. The SIDES of the wound. When the walls are undermining the viable tissue the true extent of the wound must be assessed by careful use of a sterile probe
5. The BASE of the wound for the presence of slough, granulation tissue or deeper structures such as bone or tendon. Radiographs are necessary if deeper structures are thought to be involved. The wound's DEPTH should be assessed. Chronic lesions are associated with fibrous bands tying the base to underlying structures; by gentle manipulation of the wound, the degree of fibrosis may be estimated
6. Any DISCHARGE should be noted and a specimen sent for microscopy and culture. The colour, consistency and odour of discharge should be recorded. The quantity may be approximated by observing dressings and finding out how often they require renewing.

- Disposal of soiled dressings and instruments, unless performed with care, is potentially a major source of cross-infection, and local infection-control guidelines must be followed.
- The use of instruments on any wound, and the amount of tissue debrided, will depend on the aetiology and clinical state of the lesion at the time of treatment.

Desloughing and wound-cleansing agents

Desloughing agents

Slough (a collection of necrotic material, leukocytes and micro-organisms) can become a medium for further bacterial growth; in many cases it is important to try to remove it.

Desloughing/cleansing agents include the hypochlorite group of chemicals, and enzymes that allow autolytic breakdown of slough by products generated from the patient's own leukocytes. The hypochlorites interact with protein and it is this reaction that imparts their antibacterial role. *British National Formulary* no longer recommends the use of chlorinated solutions such as Dakin's solution (Chlorinated Soda Solution, Surgical BPC) for wound cleansing due to their irritant effects.

Preparations containing enzymes are used for desloughing wounds.

Enzymes, such as streptokinase and streptodornase, are presented as dry powders, which are refrigerated until application, when they are reconstituted with sterile isotonic saline (for example, Varidase, Lederle). The solution can be held in contact with the wound using gauze and a film dressing, or it can be injected under tough necrotic slough using a syringe.

Cadexamer iodine (Iodosorb, Smith and Nephew UK) contains 0.9% w/w of iodine and exerts a hydrophilic action, acting as an absorbent. The product also helps to remove debris and bacteria from the wound surface by capillary action. The beads swell under the influence of exudate and release the iodine.

Intrasite gel can be used to help remove slough and absorb excess exudate.

Sterile larvae of *Lucilia sericata* (the common greenbottle) are used to deslough. The larvae are only 2–3 mm long when placed on the wound. They are held in situ by masking the area with a hydrocolloid sheet. The larvae are placed in a carefully shaped hole within the hydrocolloid sheet and then covered with a secondary dressing and left in situ for several days.

Wound-cleansing agents and antiseptics

The skin around the wound must be cleaned prior to treatment to reduce the number of transient micro-organisms present. Solutions of antiseptics, such as chlorhexidine gluconate in alcohol base, are satisfactory:

- chlorhexidine gluconate has activity against a wide range of both Gram-positive and Gram-negative bacteria; however, chlorhexidine is not active against fungi, spores or viruses.
- iodophors are complexes of iodine and solubilisers (for example, povidone iodine) and are found in many products, including pre-operative skin preparation.
- povidone iodine has a wide range of activity against micro-organisms, including a sporicidal action.

Wound-cleansing agents are available in sterile, single-use sachets, the use of which is strongly advocated. Solutions are applied to the wound site using sterile gauze. Cotton wool should not be used as fibres are shed onto the wound surface where they act as foreign bodies. Solutions may be applied to difficult sites via a sterile syringe barrel, without the needle attached.

Antiseptics

Most antiseptics have a deleterious effect on the wound microenvironment; they can interfere with wound healing, produce resistance in some micro-organisms and produce skin sensitivities if used for long periods of time.

The use of topical antibiotics is contraindicated; antibiotics should be delivered systemically, but only after the causative micro-organism has been identified and its sensitivity to a specific antibiotic ascertained.

Dressings

The properties of the 'ideal wound dressing' are considered before describing the various groups of products.

The criteria for the 'ideal wound dressing' are:

1. the ability to remove exudate
2. the ability to maintain humidity at the wound–dressing interface
3. permeability of the dressing to gases
4. the ability to be impermeable to micro-organisms
5. the ability to maintain a suitable temperature at the wound surface
6. the ability to maintain low adherence at the wound–dressing interface
7. the ability to be free from contaminants
8. the ability to maintain a suitable pH
9. other factors, including ease of application, patient acceptability and comfort, and cost.

> **For more information see**
> Neale's Disorders of the Foot 8E   *pages 248–249*

Types of dressing for use in podiatric practice

The introduction, and accessibility, of new dressings is changing at such a prodigious rate that a detailed description of individual dressings is inappropriate. This section will describe the features of groups of products currently available. It is stressed that before using any wound-care product practitioners should make themselves fully aware of the product's indications and contraindications, either by consulting the manufacturer or a current edition of the *British National Formulary*.

Conventional dressings

Example: Gauze swabs B.P.

- The majority of podiatrists use gauze swabs, because of availability and low cost.
- Disadvantages include: 'strike through', the shedding of fibres, adherence and incorporation into the wound surface.
- Swabs made from viscose are more absorptive and less liable to shed fibres.
- Filmated swabs have layers of cotton wool between either traditional woven, or newer non-woven gauze; this improves absorption, but can lead to shedding of fibres onto the wound surface.
- The use of paraffin gauze (the older name for which is tulle gras) reduces some of the adverse effects of using gauze; however, granulation tissue can grow through its structure and incorporate the paraffin gauze into the wound.

Primary wound-dressing films

Semipermeable adhesive film dressings

Examples: Bioclusive (Johnson & Johnson), Tegaderm (3M), Opsite (Smith & Nephew UK), Cutifilm (Beiersdorf).

They have no fibres that can be shed into wounds; they are transparent and therefore allow monitoring of the wound site. However, semipermeable adhesive films are non-absorbent.

Such dressings may be used to reduce shear stress over vulnerable areas, such as heels.

Perforated film absorbent dressings

Examples: Melolin (Smith & Nephew), Release (Johnson & Johnson).

Other low-adherence dressings incorporate an absorptive backing, covered with a perforated plastic film. Although they can absorb wound discharge, they are not suitable for heavily exuding wounds. However, a secondary absorbent dressing can be used over the top of a perforated film absorbent dressing.

Low-adherent wound contact layers

Unmedicated

Examples: N-A Dressing (Johnson & Johnson), Tricotex (Smith & Nephew).

These dressings are made from knitted viscose. They are non-absorbent but provide a non-adherent primary wound dressing.

Medicated

Examples: Bactigras (Smith & Nephew), Serotulle (Seton).

Some low-adherent wound contact dressings incorporate an antiseptic, such as chlorhexidine acetate, in a paraffin or polyethylene glycol base. Dressings with polyethylene glycol base more effectively liberate antiseptics, for example Inadine (Johnson & Johnson) which contains povidone iodine.

Semipermeable hydrogels

Example: Intrasite Gel (Smith & Nephew).

At present Intrasite Gel is the only hydrogel available on the Drug Tariff. It is composed of a low percentage of carboxy-methylcellulose, 80% water and 20% propylene glycol. Structurally these products are hydrophilic polymers that contain a high percentage of water.

Hydrocolloids

Examples: Granuflex (ConvaTec), Comfeel (Coloplast), Tegasorb (3M).

- Composed of substances that form a gel when in contact with a wound surface. Constituents adhere to, and interact with, the wound surface; these are held on a water-repellent, flexible, foam backing, which should not require a secondary dressing.
- The occlusive environment contraindicates the use of hydrocolloids when a wound is clinically infected – particularly when anaerobe species are isolated. The use of hydrocolloids may also be contraindicated for treating diabetic ulcers.
- Hydrocolloids are available in other presentations (for example pastes); these are used in wounds supporting a heavy slough. Most manufacturers produce 'wound-management systems'; these involve using desloughing agents, and specific types of dressing at different stages of wound healing.

Alginate dressings

Examples: Kaltostat (BritCair ConvaTec), Sorbsan (Maersk).

These products are manufactured from calcium and sodium salts of alginic acid, derived from seaweed. They represent a very old treatment: sailors used seaweed for dressing wounds and effecting haemostasis centuries ago.

Generally, alginates are relatively easy to remove, provided that the area is irrigated with sterile isotonic saline; however, some situations will require the use of forceps to complete the removal of the dressing. Theoretically, the fibres associated with the dressing present no hazard as they are biodegradable.

Polyurethane foams

Examples: Lyofoam (Seton), Allevyn (Smith & Nephew).

Foams are indicated for treating wounds with moderate amounts of exudate.

Foam dressings are very permeable to gases and allow adequate hydration of the wound surface. They also provide effective thermal insulation.

Silver agents

Silver-impregnated dressings are a recent introduction. Silver is known to be antibacterial.

Other aspects of management

- Education and advice about preventing secondary complications of the disease is imperative and part of the podiatric management.
- The use of padding and orthoses to protect wounds may be indicated; each patient will require a specific prescription, therefore only general comments can be made.
- Soft cushioning padding materials will be indicated rather than firm redistributive materials.
- Accurate positioning of pads is vital.
- As little adhesive as practically possible should be placed on the skin; the use of conforming bandages for example, Kling (Johnson & Johnson) or plastic film sprays can be used to protect vulnerable areas of skin from adhesives.
- Replaceable silicone pads (Silipos) of various shapes and sizes are useful.
- When specific areas of high-pressure loading are identified, casted insoles constructed from composites of low-, medium- and high-density thermoplastics may be required.
- Footwear and hosiery must be carefully selected and, if necessary, modifications such as stretching or balloon patching can be executed.
- Slippers, often a popular choice with patients, are not recommended unless well fitting, as they produce shearing stresses that cause movement of dressings, predispose to falls and reduce activity of the calf muscle pump.
- Total contact casting may be indicated when treating neuropathic ulcers. The technique must be taught correctly from someone with experience in the technique, and the podiatrist must be confident in the correct application of the cast before attempting to use total contact casts on patients.
- The introduction of Aircast pneumatic walkers has proved beneficial for some patients; these transfer pressure over the whole of the plantar surface of the feet and support the leg, and they also have a rocker sole. When these methods are used the patient must be provided with an address or telephone number that they may access 24 hours a day, 7 days a week, in case advice is needed.
- Rest and elevate the affected limb, but the danger of immobility producing a deep-vein thrombosis cannot be overlooked. Other problems of immobility are the development of pressure sores and, if the limb is insufficiently elevated, oedema may ensue.
- Patients must be discouraged from smoking.
- Patient's quality of life, and their compliance, may be adversely affected unless compromise between ideal and realistic advice is given.

- When wounds develop they must be treated on an individual basis, and only after a full medical history and physical examination of the patient, and their lesion, have been carried out. When selecting wound-care products the practitioner is aided by an understanding of the normal wound-healing process and by frequent consultation of the medical and nursing press for new developments.

Chapter | **11** |

Podiatric management
of the elderly

Life expectancy has increased dramatically over the last century. These improvements have resulted in an increasingly ageing population, with similar findings repeated across all developed countries.

A variety of conditions may affect the elderly, these may be conditions that are specifically associated with ageing or conditions that may affect a range of age groups, but may become more complicated in the elderly patient.

NAIL CONDITIONS AND CARE

A range of nail conditions present in older people, however, the most common include:

- onychauxis
- onychogryphosis
- onychomycosis.

ADDITIONAL PROBLEMS

- Subungual helomata
- Hyperextension of the hallux in hallux limitus/rigidus
- Overlapping of the toes in hallux abductovalgus
- Onychophosis
- Paronychia and onychia. There may be an increased risk of opportunistic infections which may manifest as:
  - cellulitis
  - tissue breakdown
  - ulceration and bacteraemia
- Repeated minor trauma or undue pressure to a thickened toenail from footwear may produce:
  - non-infected sub-ungual breakdown
  - sub-ungual ulceration.
- To prevent such a condition occurring the podiatrist must ensure that the thickened nail is skilfully reduced.

ENVIRONMENTAL FACTORS AFFECTING THE FOOT

- *Maceration* of the skin occurs when the normal regulation of skin water content is disturbed, this may be:
  - intrinsic because of excessive sweating
  - extrinsic when evaporation of moisture cannot take place
- Older patients sometimes find it difficult to carry out usual foot hygiene and fail to dry properly. Un-treated, the skin may:
  - split to form painful fissures and/or ulceration
  - increase the risk of colonisation by bacteria or fungi
  - go on to frank infection either as erythrasma, a yeast infection or tinea pedis.

RISK FACTORS ASSOCIATED WITH THE DEVELOPMENT OF ULCERATION IN THE FEET AND LEGS

- Venous leg ulcers affect between 0.15 and 0.8% of the population
- Venous hypertension leads to:
  - capillary distortion
  - increased capillary permeability.

  This leads to the classic signs of:

- haemosiderin deposits
- venous eczema
- lipodermatosclerosis.

The treatment of ulceration may require the skills and knowledge of a variety of healthcare professionals:

- podiatrist
- dietician
- district nurse
- vascular specialist.

HOLISTIC CARE

Musculoskeletal changes

There are a number of physiological changes that occur as a normal consequence of the ageing process. These include changes to:

- the integumentary system
- peripheral vascular system
- musculoskeletal system.

Muscle tissue

- Age-related change in muscle fibre mass is known as sarcopenia, or senile sarcopenia.

Table 11.1 Ulcer healing

NUTRITIONAL PREREQUISITES FOR OPTIMAL WOUND HEALING	POSITIVE EFFECTS ON ULCER HEALING
Carbohydrates	Energy for fibroblast and leukocyte function
Protein	Phagocytosis Angiogenesis Collagen synthesis Wound remodelling
Vitamin A, C, B12 complex	Collagen synthesis Macrophage migration Epithelialisation
Vitamin K	Clotting cascade
Zinc Manganese Copper Magnesium	Cell division Epithelialisation Collagen strengthening

- Muscle mass reduction is thought to decrease by approx 40% between the ages of 20 and 60.
- Maximum contractile strength is thought to decrease by 20–40% for both men and women in advancing age in both proximal and distal muscles.
- In cases where co-morbidities and reduced activity levels co-exist, the rate at which sarcopenia occurs is thought to significantly increase.

Tendon and ligament

- Collagen type 1 is the main type of collagen present in tendons and ligaments.
- It is thought that there is a general decline in older age of the number of tenocytes present and, therefore, the reparative process may take longer.
- Research has demonstrated that some tendons, for example the posterior tibial tendon, are more susceptible to damage in the older age group.

Management of change

- There is clear evidence that exercise and muscle-strengthening programmes prescribed to older people can have a positive effect on muscle strength.
- Balance is a significant risk factor for falls. Foot and ankle characteristics are significantly related to balance and functional ability in older people.
- Nutritional intake of proteins and vitamins, particularly vitamin C, is also thought to be important (Table 11.1). Additional protein intake by the way of supplements may have a positive benefit on muscle mass.
- Exercise and correct nutrition in older people, may help prevent the adverse effects of senescent sarcopenia.

FALLS IN OLDER PEOPLE

Risk factors associated with falls

- Falls are not an inevitable consequence of ageing. It is in the identification of risk and the subsequent management of those risk factors that can help in falls prevention.
- Non-injurious fall is often a precursor to a more serious injurious fall, and can often lead to psychological sequelae leading to:
  - a fear of further falls
  - restricted mobility
  - social isolation which in turn leads to further risk of falling.
- The risk factors identified in the NICE guidelines (2004) include:
  - poor balance
  - visual impairment
  - Parkinsonism
  - stroke
  - gait abnormalities
  - use of assist devices
  - depression
  - cognitive impairment
  - environmental factors
  - mobility impairment
  - reduced activity
  - poly-pharmacy
  - muscle weakness
  - low body mass, arthritis
  - impaired activities of daily living
  - high alcohol consumption.

Falls risk assessment

- To identify whether a patient may be at risk of falls through motor strength deficits affecting mobility, the 'get up and go' test provides a useful indicator.

Inappropriate footwear

- Shoe style is thought to be a significant factor in respect of falls often associated with:
  - elevated heel height
  - heavy boots
  - boots with a cut-away heel
- An investigation into the footwear worn at the time of a falls-related hip fracture revealed that slippers were the most prevalent shoe style.

The ideal footwear style for an older person

The evidence suggests that the key features to consider are:

- tread of the sole of the shoe
- heel height.

Many older people do not base their footwear selection on the premise of safety and rather base their choices entirely on comfort. However, footwear deemed most comfortable has been associated with a shoe that gives a high balance failure

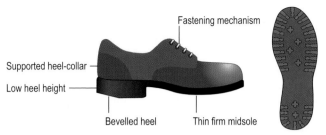

Figure 11.1 Recommended characteristics of shoe style for older people. *Menant et al, 2008. Optimizing Footwear for older people at risk of falls. Journal of Rehabilitation Research and Development. 48(8):1167–1181.*

rate. The advice needs to take into account the holistic picture of individual circumstance and may include:

- environmental factors
- psychosocial factors
- medical and surgical history
- personal circumstances.

Recommended characteristics of shoe style – see Figure 11.1

Poly pharmacy

- Patients taking more than three or four medications are considered to be at risk of recurrent falls.
- Certain drugs are thought to be risk-increasing drugs, and should be considered as part of a falls risk assessment, these drugs, include:
  - sulphonamides and potassium-sparing diuretics
  - hypnotics
  - calcium preparations
  - central acting obesity products
  - bioflavonoids.

Long-term disease and older people

- Circulatory disease, chronic obstructive pulmonary disease, depression, and arthritis were each associated with higher odds of falling.

QUALITY OF LIFE

- Many elderly individuals live independently with a number of chronic conditions that cause difficulty in a number of areas of daily life affecting their ability to perform and maintain activities of daily living (ADLs).
- Healthcare practitioners should be sensitive to the fact that older people can have a range of related conditions that can have a significant impact on their ability to remain independent and maintain a quality of life that they deserve.
- A report indicated that there was a much higher incidence of disability when more than one chronic disease was present:
  - 50% reported difficulty with mobility
  - 35% reported difficulty with upper extremity tasks
  - 22% with self-care tasks
  - 22% with higher functioning household tasks.

- The study also showed that when diseases were paired there was a reoccurrence with specific pairings that was consistently affecting mobility. These included: OA and high blood pressure, joint arthritis and visual problems, heart disease and cancer, and stroke and high blood pressure. Ranked eighth were arthritis and hearing impairment.

Duty of care

- As part of the multidisciplinary health and social care workforce podiatrists are required to work within the Codes of Conduct for Podiatrists as set out by the Professional Regulator, in the case of the United Kingdom is the Health Professions Council.
- Most podiatrists are also members of a professional body and members are expected to abide by their Code of Conduct or Ethics.
- The greatest challenge for the podiatrist is to guide the patient into deciding to seek help from outside the family. Some older patients may:
  - be reluctant to seek help
  - be ignorant of the eligibility criteria, and the nature and extent of services available
  - declare themselves to be coping adequately.
- The healthcare professional has a responsibility to provide information to patients and clients in order to improve health, prevent illness and, importantly, enable them to maintain their independence.
- Sensitive, well-developed communication skills are required when discussing these issues with both patients and carers, as this sort of information provision may be seen to imply criticism of the patients:
  - living arrangements
  - self-care ability.

Hypothermia risk

Accidental hypothermia is an unintentional drop in temperature and is suffered by the elderly. The older individual is particularly susceptible to hypothermia as there is both a decrease in heat generation and at the same time an increase in heat loss. Generation of heat results from muscle activity and decreases in the elderly primarily as a consequence of:

- a 30% reduction of muscle bulk in people 70 years old
- a reduction in activity levels by as much as a 50%.

  Other risk factors include:

- inadequate clothing
- poor nutrition
- depressant drugs
- alcohol
- systemic conditions such as hypothyroidism and diabetes.

Dehydration

Dehydration is a common finding in the elderly population. The symptoms are insidious and non-specific and include:

- lassitude
- fatigue
- muscle cramps
- dizziness caused by postural hypotension.

Thirst decreases with age and with the normal ageing of the kidneys that results in a reduced ability to concentrate urine the condition is exacerbated. At the same time, urine flow is generally maintained resulting in further dehydration. Dehydration may also be caused by the use of:

- potent dieuretics
- antipsychotics
- sedatives
- non-steroidal anti-inflammatory drugs (NSAIDs).

Further risk factors include:

- incontinence
- lack of mobility
- dementia
- consumption of alcohol and caffeine drinks.

The possible consequences of dehydration for the elderly are serious and include:

- urinary tract infection
- bowel obstruction
- delirium
- cardiovascular symptoms
- death.

A study listed key risk factors which should alert the healthcare professional to the possibility of dehydration. These factors include:

- being female
- being over 85 years old
- having four or more chronic medical conditions
- taking four or more medications
- being confined to bed
- using laxatives inappropriately
- suffering chronic infection (Bennett 2000).

Such patients should be considered at risk of dehydration and advice should include encouragement to take plenty of water, fruit drinks or non-salty soups.

Dementia and depression

Mental health problems are suffered by 25% of the elderly population and include depression and anxiety. Dementia affects some 10% of the over 65 age group rising to 20% in those over 80 years old.

The dementias are a group of diseases defined by clinical cognitive deficits including:

- memory impairment
- an inability to recall previous information or to learn new information
- aphasia
- apraxia
- agnosia
- disturbances in executive functioning, such as planning, organising, etc.

There are many causes of dementia including metabolic disorders and neurological conditions; however, 70% of cases are caused by Alzheimer's disease.

Alzheimer's is not only devastating for the patient but also to the family and carers. In addition there is a considerable cost burden on society for residential care or for support to enable the patient to remain in their own home.

Depression affects between 1% and 4% of the general elderly population, with twice as many women than men affected. Prevalence and incidence rates double after the age of 70–85. Prevalence of minor depression in the elderly is between 4 and 13% and very old people are especially prone to this condition. Individuals in residential homes suffer greater rates of all types of depression than those who remain living in the community.

The key signs for three types of depressive disorder are:

- *major depressive disorder* – depressed mood, diminished interest, loss of pleasure in almost all activities, weight loss or gain, insomnia, agitation, fatigue, feelings of worthlessness, inappropriate guilt, recurrent thoughts of death or suicide.
- *minor depressive disorder* – at least two of the above symptoms must be present for at least 2 weeks and lead to distress and impaired function which cannot be attributed to a medical condition or bereavement.
- *dysthymic disorder* – a chronic condition characterised by a sad mood that occurs for most of the day, more days than not, for at least 2 years. The condition is diagnosed if accompanied by two symptoms of major depressive disorder.

The elderly may suffer depression that is associated with:

- viral infection
- endocrine disorders of thyroid parathyroid adrenal glands
- malignancy, leukaemia, pancreatic cancer
- cerebro-vascular disease such as stroke, vascular dementia
- myocardial infarction
- metabolic disorder – malnutrition vitamin B12 deficiency.

They may also exhibit symptoms associated with the use or cessation of use of:

- anti-parkinsonism drugs
- beta blockers
- tamoxifen
- benzodiazepines
- propanolol
- reserpine
- steroids.

The management aims for depression are:

- to reduce distressing symptoms
- to prevent relapse
- to improve cognitive function.

Importantly patients should be helped to develop skills to cope with their disability or psychosocial difficulties.

Osteoporosis and fracture

This is characterised by low bone mass and deterioration of bone tissue and leads to increased bone fragility and increased risk of fracture (Consensus development conference 1993). Foot and ankle fractures are among the most common non-spinal fractures occurring in the elderly. One study found that fracture of the 5th metatarsal was the most common foot fracture in osteoporosis sufferers.

Risk factors for osteoporosis

- Advanced age
- Previous low-trauma fracture
- Low body mass index
- Smoking

- Glucocorticoids
- Excessive alcohol consumption
- Rheumatoid arthritis
- Parental fracture.

Incontinence

Urinary incontinence or enuresis is common in the elderly and is distressing and disabling. Elderly individuals with dementia are more likely to be incontinent than those with normal mental function.

Other causes of incontinence in the older person whose mobility is impaired include:

- potent diuretics
- constipation
- infection.

Malnutrition

Between the ages of 20 and 80 years there is a gradual reduction in the amount of food that people eat (Wakimoto & Block 2001). To eat less food as a response to decreased activity is appropriate, however, in some cases a reduction in food intake may place the older person at risk of a pathological weight loss if accompanied by chronic disease known as 'anorexia of ageing' (Wilson & Morley 2003).

Malnutrition in the older population has also been associated with:

- increased hospital stay
- discharge destination
- infections, gait disorders
- falls
- fractures
- pressure sores and poor wound healing.

A study indicated that factors that may lead a clinician to suspect the patient may be malnourished are:

- poor oral health with red sebborrheic nasolabila folds
- lax, pale dry skin with loss of turgor and pigmented patches
- thinning or loss of hair
- diminished sensory function
- thirst
- nocturia
- diminished tendon jerks
- subnormal body temperature.

Chapter | **12** |

Paediatric podiatry and genetics

This differs from the role of other sectors of podiatry as there is an opportunity to prevent and correct deformity and maintain normal function, underpinned by footwear prescription and advice and health promotion as part of a multidisciplinary team.

Traditional skills in the management of skin, soft-tissue lesions, nail conditions and infections are still necessary but play a smaller part. Monitoring, charting and advising over time are the main requirements.

When dealing with structural problems the practitioner must always be satisfied that they are dealing with a pathological state requiring intervention and not a 'normal' variant of developmental change.

NORMAL GROWTH AND DEVELOPMENT

The majority of children are born with normal feet. The shape, size and form of feet are genetically determined but are affected by other factors. The conditions present at birth are designated congenital disorders.

Ossification starts in the larger bones of the foot and leg extending to the smaller bones (Table 12.1).

The child's foot is not a small-scale replica of the adult foot:

- it is shorter and wider, tapering towards the heel.
- the infant's foot is malleable and allows some congenital deformities to be corrected easily.
- the foot appears short, broad, stubby-toed and fat at birth.
- it appears flat due to fatty padding in the medial longitudinal arch area, but this is gradually absorbed as growth proceeds.
- constrictive foot coverings should be avoided to allow normal growth and development. It is important to allow freedom of movement for muscle development.

Table 12.1 Ossification timetable

BONE	PRIMARY CENTRES	SECONDARY CENTRES	FUSION REMARKS
Tibia – diaphysis	7th week		
Tibia – upper epiphysis	At birth	20th year	
Tibia – lower epihysis	2nd year	18th year	Sometimes a separate centre for the medial malleolus appears at the same time
Fibula – diaphysis	8th week		
Fibula – upper epiphysis		4th year	25th year
Fibula – lower epiphysis		2nd year	20th year
Calcaneus – body	6th month		
Calcaneus – epiphysis	6th–10th month		13th–15th year
Talus	7th month		
Cuboid	At birth		
Lateral cuneiform	1st year		
Medial cuneiform	3rd year		
Intermediate cuneiform	4th year		
Navicular	4th year		
1st metatarsal shaft	8th–9th week		
1st metatarsal base	3rd year	17th–20th year	Sometimes a separate centre for the head appears at the same time
Other metatarsal shafts	8th–9th week		Sometimes a separate centre for the base of the 5th metatarsal appears at the same time
Proximal phalanx shafts	12th–14th weeks		
Proximal phalanx bases	3rd–6th years	17th–18th years	
Intermediate phalanx shafts	4th–9th month		That for the 5th toe does not appear until shortly after birth

BONE	PRIMARY CENTRES	SECONDARY CENTRES	FUSION REMARKS
Intermediate phalanx bases distal phalanx of hallux		3rd–6th year	17th–18th year
Distal phalanx shafts	8th week		
Distal phalanx bases		6th year	17th–18th year

Table 12.1 Ossification timetable—cont'd

- during the crawling and walking stages bare-footed walking is best to encourage normal function.
- it is best that children do not wear shoes until they are walking competently out of doors.

Gait and general posture constantly change in the developing child. Knock knees and a flat foot are normal at specific stages in development.

- A young child walks on a broad base, appears flat-footed with bow legs, exhibits lordosis, bulging of the abdomen and legs partly flexed at the knees.
- The feet may be variously abducted or adducted and apparently 'flat'.
- From 2 to 6 years of age, developmental knock-knee is evident and should resolve around age 5–6.
- Foot type and medial longitudinal arch become more evident around 6 years of age.
- Developmental changes in the lower limb result in compensation of subtalar joint pronation.
- Older children very frequently have flattening of the medial longitudinal arch on standing but the arch reasserts itself on standing on tiptoe.

Peak rates of growth

- Accelerated growth in girls occurs between 8 and 13 peaking at 12 years of age.
- Accelerated growth in boys occurs between 10.5 and 16 peaking at 14 years of age.
- Many foot pathologies seen in children in this age group are associated with growth.
- This age group tends to be more active, putting additional stress on growing tissues.
- Children under the management of a podiatrist should have their feet and height measured and charted at each visit.
- Growth rate of feet is constant from birth, increasing by approximately two sizes per year for the first 4 years and then by one size annually thereafter until the mid-teens.

FOOTWEAR

Children's footwear presents in many forms and should be examined and its suitability considered with every patient. Hazards include:

- babygros and sleep suits. Made from cotton, washing may reduce their size
- stretch tights and socks. Attention is paid to shoe fitting, hosiery is often neglected and inadequate hosiery damages the growing foot
- knitted booties with an open weave can result in entrapment of a digit and resultant gangrene due to ischaemia and are often badly fitting
- pram shoes. Permanent use should be discouraged due to sizing and fitting difficulties. Synthetic materials are unsuitable, encouraging excessive sweating.

Exceptions include:

- children born with deformity such as talipes equinovarus or neurological conditions such as hemiplegia when the foot must be maintained in a corrected position. In these circumstances the footwear would be prescribed professionally.

Inadequate footwear

Footwear may be inadequate in several ways, including:

- too short
- too narrow
- pointed or a shallow toe box
- poor or no retaining medium
- inadequate heel stiffener
- heel height too high
- narrow base to the heel
- synthetic uppers and/or lining
- not compatible with the foot.

Children should always have the feet measured for shoes by a trained competent shoe fitter. Feet should be measured at approximately 2-month intervals and the shoes replaced as required.

Plimsolls

- Some schools require plimsolls to be worn in school all day. Problems are:
  - plimsolls are placed in shoe bags overnight
  - they do not dry out fully and are worn again the next day
  - good fitting shoes which have been purchased carefully are hardly worn
  - the plimsolls which remain at school are not replaced timeously as the foot grows
  - the growing foot may be in an unhealthy damp environment
  - plimsolls are not fitted accurately and are often too small
  - plimsolls are excellent only for the purpose for which they are intended, i.e. gymnastics
  - they do not provide a suitable environment for a growing foot
  - plimsolls do not allow for the changing flare of a young foot
  - they are unsuitable as a vehicle for casted orthoses.

Children walk at differing ages and it is best to 'let nature take its course' and allow the child to walk when ready rather than prematurely stressing tissues and loading joints with the use of babywalkers.

It is important to recognise when managing the case of the teenager that compromises regarding footwear have to be made with regard to:

- fashion trends
- peer group pressure
- economics.

Communicate with teenagers at a different level and understand and advise them accordingly.

Trainers

- Good so long as the criteria for an adequate footwear is followed
- If made from synthetic material poor ventilation and absorption of sweat predispose the foot to verrucae, tinea pedis and onychocryptosis.

FOOT TYPE

Foot types are many and varied, therefore, footwear should be fitted by an experienced, competent fitter with a wide range of styles, sizes and fittings.

- The infant foot is triangular in shape
- As the child progresses into adolescence shape becomes rectangular
- A child's shoe is in-flared and an adults relatively straight-flared by comparison
- The 1st ray is in a relatively adducted position and a straight-flared or small shoe may cause soft-tissue pathologies or digital deformity.

Typical foot types include:

- short broad
- square forefoot
- hypermobile
- long slender
- triangular
- long inner border
- low arched
- high arched.

INFECTIONS

Infections are most commonly bacterial, fungal or viral. The most common 'paediatric foot' infections are:

- tinea pedis
- verrucae
- onychocryptosis
- paronychia
- infections from foreign bodies
- infected blisters.

These conditions can occur at any age, but are most common among teenagers and children who are immunocompromised (undergoing chemotherapy) or those with lymphoedema (Turner's syndrome) where there is an added risk of cellulitis.

ANATOMICAL ANOMALIES

These include:

- sesamoid bones, supernumerary bones
- os trigonum, os tibial externum and os vesalii
- tarsal coalition (peroneal spastic flat foot). Calcaneo-navicular coalition, fusion occurs across the midtarsal joint. Talocalcaneal coalition, fusion occurs between the sustentaculum tali and the talus:
  - may be symptomless
  - may have distressing painful symptoms making surgery necessary
  - may present with painful contraction of the peroneal muscles resulting in a fixed, everted, abducted foot as the result of a growth spurt – a 'spastic flat foot' develops:
    - examination reveals tender, taut and prominent peroneal tendons and attempts to invert the foot will be painfully resisted
    - specialist X-rays and/or a CT scan may be necessary to demonstrate the fusion
    - initial therapy is resting the foot in a below-knee plaster cast
    - surgery for recurrent or intractable pain
    - long-term follow-up management with casted foot orthoses.

BIOMECHANICAL ANOMALIES/ABNORMALITIES

Acquired deformity

Virtually any pathology is possible but the most common are digital deformities including:

- hammer toe
- mallet toe
- retracted toe
- claw toe
- varus position of the toes
- hallux abductovalgus
- serious forefoot disruption and deformity due to excessive subtalar joint (STJ) pronation.

Juvenile hallux abductovalgus

Aetiology

- Footwear
- A strong family history
- Excessive abnormal STJ pronation.

Treatment

- Footwear advice
- Exercises
- Silicone devices – inter-digital wedges incorporated with a two to four combined prop in order to splint the hallux against the lesser toes and thus promote correction

- Orthoses
- Night splints should be used in conjunction with exercises and orthotic management
- Review at 6-weekly intervals if attempting correction.

Juvenile hallux rigidus

Aetiology

- Uncommon in children
- Usually teenage males
- Recurrent minor trauma
- Single incident
- Produces a chondral injury
- Pain and muscle spasm results in loss of extension at the metatarsophalangeal joint
- Patient walks on the outer border of the foot to avoid the painful area
- Rest in a cast is the first-line treatment
- Proximal phalangeal osteotomy when symptoms persist:
  - Treatment:
    - appropriate physical therapy
    - padding and strapping
    - footwear advice.

The lower limbs

Examination of the musculoskeletal system should commence with:

- observation of the infant or child in static stance and gait
- observation of limb position
- inspection of the lower limbs of an infant for signs of dissimilarity in:
  - the skin creases
  - girth
  - gross abnormalities such as bowing of the legs
  - discrepancy in leg length – usually due to:
    - muscle wasting
    - poor development
    - neurological problem
    - larger limb abnormal due to hypertrophy, lymphoedema or malformation.

Digital abnormalities

- Polydactyly – supernumerary digits attached either to the hand or the foot
- Syndactyly (webbed toes – zygodactyly) – a total or partial fusion of adjacent digits
- Oligodactyly – the developmental absence of one or more of all metatarsal parts and phalanges
- Congenital overlapping 5th toe (digiti minimi quinti varus) – from birth the toe lies on the dorsum of the base of the 4th toe in a medially deviated position. This is the only common toe abnormality in childhood to need surgical correction
- Curly toes – are common, bilateral or unilateral. The 4th and 5th are flexed and curled medially. If the 3rd is flexed with medial deformity, the 2nd is deformed, lies on a higher plane and curls laterally, overlying the 3rd toe
- Congenital flexed toe – is uncommon and may affect one toe or two adjacent toes

- Metatarsus adductus – less common deformity – the forefoot is deviated towards the midline in relation to the hindfoot. This is treated early with serial well-padded moulded plasters
- Hallux varus – an uncommon condition – seen with metatarsus adductus, frequently corrects with growth. Occasionally surgery is required.

CONGENITAL DEFORMITIES

Talipes equinovarus: clubfoot

This common deformity occurs 2–4 times in every thousand births.

Diagnosis

- On inspection the deformity is in three parts:
  - the heel is drawn up
  - the foot is inverted
  - the hindfoot is adducted
  - a minority have a postural deformity which is corrected easily by manipulation to neutral and beyond
  - the majority have rigidly deformed feet
  - clubfoot deformities are also found in arthrogryposis, trisomy 18 and spina bifida cystica.

Treatment

- Daily manipulation of each element of the deformity
- Correction obtained each day is maintained with application of a Denis Browne splint
- As the deformity improves the splint is bent to hold a greater degree of correction and then connected to the other foot
- Over a period of 7–14 days the foot will reach the overcorrected position
- Overcorrection is maintained by re-manipulation and re-application of the splints every 2 weeks until the child learns to stand
- Alternatively the corrected position is maintained by the use of Elastoplast strapping or plaster of Paris
- For walking, the splints are discarded and boots with an outer raise to the sole are used with night boots and corrective bar for bed
- Parents use manipulation to hold the foot in overcorrected position
- Gradually treatments can be abandoned with a view to the child going to school at 5 years of age with normal footwear
- Soft-tissue release operation on the medial and posterior aspects of the foot and ankle is needed if the foot is inadequately corrected during the first year or relapses in later years
- About half of the corrected feet require this procedure
- Foot orthoses with life-long podiatric management may be required.

Talipes calcaneovalgus

This is the opposite deformity from clubfoot:

- usually the result of *in utero* posture
- prognosis is excellent as natural improvement occurs with active movement on leaving the uterus

- the deformity resolves permanently within weeks with manipulation of the foot into equinovarus frequently by the parent
- condition is less commonly associated with congenital dislocation of the hip and tibial deformity.

Vertical talus (rocker bottom foot)

This is a rare deformity caused by a dislocation of the talonavicular joint and it occurs in 10–50% of patients with trisomy 18 syndrome.

Treatment

- Surgical correction to reduce the dislocation of the talonavicular joint
- In the older child bony correction or fusion will be needed
- Foot orthoses may be required to maintain foot posture.

Onychogryphosis

Often thought of as an acquired complaint of the elderly, this condition can be congenital – affecting any toe or toes, but usually the 1st or 5th. It is easily managed conservatively.

Arthrogryposis multiplex congenita

This is a congenital condition affecting joints:
- may be localised or generalised
- joints may be extended or flexed
- a severe degree of talipes is present
- muscles are atrophic and fibrous
- skin is tight – the limbs resemble hosepipes
- arthroplasty fails to provide useful movement
- treatment is to stabilise the affected joints in good position.

Congenital constriction band syndrome

- May result in congenital absence of toes
- Condition occurs *in utero*
- Can result in amputation of the part if it occurs in early foetal life
- Presents as ring-like concentric bands which may be deep or shallow
- Deep bands affect lymphatic and venous drainage resulting in oedema.

SURGICAL/MEDICAL CONDITIONS

Leg-length discrepancy

- Up to 1 cm difference in true length is considered a normal variation
- Causes a compensatory pelvic tilt and secondary spinal scoliosis
- The child may 'toe walk' to lengthen the leg
- Adoptive shortening of the Achilles tendon
- Imposes abnormal stresses on the talus, changes the function and structure of the foot with growth
- Leg-length discrepancy may develop due to a variety of causes:
  - rare events, such as arteriovenous malformation
  - following acute osteitis

- shortening due to mal-union of a fracture
- progressive shortening when epiphyseal growth plates are damaged
- poliomyelitis can result in severe leg-length discrepancy
- Less than 3 cm is accommodated by a shoe or heel raise
- Deficiencies greater than 3 cm may be dealt with by:
  - shortening of the longer leg
  - retarding growth in the longer leg by destroying or stapling the epiphyseal plates
  - lengthening the short leg.

Linear scleroderma

This is a linear band of hypopigmentation and sclerosis:

- legs are most commonly involved usually unilateral distribution
- growth failure affects the limb due to atrophy of muscle and skin affecting bone development.

Localised scleroderma (morphea)

- More common than systemic form
- Morphea begins as a circumscribed patch of skin induration
- Typically on the trunk or feet
- At onset skin is oedematous and warm and characteristically has a violaceous border with an ivory centre
- Range of joint motion limited.

Pes cavus

- Wide variation in arch height
- Can be uni- or bilateral
- Affected leg is thinner and shorter
- Foot is often smaller
- Develops in the early years
- May have a neurological cause due to minor anomalies in the lumbosacral cord region.

Investigations

- Myelography
- Magnetic resonance imaging
- Direct surgical exploration.

Treatment

- Podiatric management.

Osteochondrosis

Sever's disease (calcaneal apophysitis)

- Affects 10–14-year-olds
- Pain at the point of the heel
- Worse during or after activity
- Calcaneal apophysis is tender at heel strike
- Pain on tiptoe
- 50% affected are bilateral.

Diagnosis

This is dependent on:

- history
- tenderness about the point of the heel
- X-rays are normal.

Treatment

- Restrict activity
- Cycling and swimming are alternatives to football or netball
- Absorbent rubber heel pad to the shoe
- Affected foot should always be investigated for forefoot/hindfoot malalignment
- Appropriate foot orthoses
- Very active children may present with Sever's disease, Osgood–Schlatter's disease and pain at the insertion of the plantar fascia which is treated with rest and appropriate foot orthoses.

Kohler's disease of the navicular

- Affects the navicular bone
- Causes vague pain about the midfoot
- Tender locally
- X-ray findings show increased density and collapse of the navicular
- Minimal treatment by supportive padding and strapping or casted supportive foot orthoses
- X-ray appearances normal in 1 to 2 years.

Freiberg's disease

- Affects the epiphysis of the 2nd, occasionally the 3rd metatarsal
- X-rays show an irregular increase in density and flattening of the metatarsal
- Develops a large square-shaped metatarsal head.

Treatment

- May require excision in adulthood
- Protect the area with appropriate padding and strapping in childhood
- The use of 1–5 PMP with 'U's, 2–4 PMPs, props or dorsoplantar splints
- Forefoot/rearfoot malalignment is managed with orthoses.

Stress fracture of a metatarsal (march or fatigue fracture)

- Increase in physical activity may stress a metatarsal
- Undisplaced self-healing fracture
- Local pain, tenderness and swelling
- Moderate rest with supportive padding and strapping
- Orthotic device
- A walking plaster is required in some cases.

Diabetes

Currently, the incidence of diabetes among children in the general population in Scotland is 25 per 100 000 and in England 13 per 100 000. Children with diabetes do not require any specialist podiatric care different to other children so long as they are controlled and free from acquired foot infections. It is important that all diabetic children are screened by the podiatrist at yearly intervals:

- to detect and manage any digital deformities
- assess and manage biomechanical disorders
- reduce the risk from pressure lesions that may occur
- provide appropriate health education.

Spina bifida cystica

- Sacral lesions lead to foot problems
- Sensory loss may be extensive
- Motor dysfunction due to root damage results in flaccid paralysis
- Areas of spasticity may be present due to higher cord damage with intact lower cord with a potential to develop severe deformity
- A common level of lesion at L4 will leave the roots of femoral and obturator nerves largely intact while the sciatic nerve will be paralysed. The hip, subject to the pull of flexors and adductors but with no extensor or abductor muscle function, will dislocate
- Active quadriceps, unopposed by paralysed hamstrings, will produce recurvatum of the knee
- The foot may be deformed in any direction and the loss of the normal weight distribution on the sole of the foot will readily lead to trophic ulceration in the anaesthetic foot.

Treatment

- Leg deformity may be controlled and function improved by calliper bracing
- Success in getting the child to stand or walk with various aids depend on:
  - the child's intelligence
  - the degree of neurological damage
  - the possible presence of spinal deformity
- Obesity should be controlled to make standing and walking easier
- A wheelchair existence is the likely result in many children
- Avoid ill-fitting appliances or footwear. Sensory loss leads to:
  - trophic ulceration, which must be treated rigourously
- Children with spina bifida should be regularly monitored by a podiatrist and treated, referred or advised as circumstances dictate.

Cerebral palsy

- Denotes a disorder of movement
- The spastic group shows the features of muscle spasm resulting in spastic postures of the limb
- The most common is spastic tetraplegia in which all four limbs are involved:
  - This group is subdivided into types I and II:
    - type I spastic tetraplegia – the legs are more severely involved than the arms
    - type II spastic tetraplegia – the spasticity is extremely severe in all four limbs
- A team approach to management of all modalities of therapy is required
- Inevitably for the podiatrist foot care may become a primary treatment.

Muscular dystrophies

This comprises a group of genetically determined disorders with a common denominator of a progressive degenerative process in the skeletal muscles. Many of these children later develop foot problems and may require help from a podiatrist.

Hypermobility syndrome

Generalised joint laxity is a feature of the hereditary connective tissue disorders such as Marfan's syndrome, the Ehlers–Danlos syndrome and osteogenesis imperfecta. Hypermobility is present if two of the following three manoeuvres are present:

- passive opposition of both thumbs to the volar aspect of the forearms
- passive hyperextension of the fingers so they lie parallel to the extensor aspect of both forearms
- active hyperextension of both elbows beyond 180°.

Casted foot orthoses may be of benefit during acute episodes and in maintaining foot posture.

Limb pain of childhood with no organic disease

So-called 'limb pains' or 'growing pains' are more common in childhood than all the other rheumatic diseases put together.

- Growth in children involves two phases – 'shooting up' and 'filling out'.
- A limb may show bone growth followed by (not accompanied by) muscle growth.
- Extra strain is on the muscle which tires easily and gives pain.
- Two-thirds have limb pains during the daytime or evening.
- One-third has nocturnal pain.
- The age group is 9–12 years – girls more than boys.
- The pain is muscular.
- Most children find gentle rubbing eases the pain.
- Occasionally, children have psychosomatic musculoskeletal pain and should have a full psychological evaluation.
- Foot orthoses are of use in some cases, particularly where there is an obvious biomechanical abnormality.

Juvenile idiopathic arthritis (juvenile chronic arthritis)

Juvenile idiopathic arthritis comprises a heterogeneous group.

- It may present as:
  - oligoarthritis
  - systemic arthritis
  - polyarthritis (rheumatoid factor-(RF)-negative antinuclear antibody-(ANA)-positive)
  - polyarthritis (RF-negative, ANA-negative)
  - polyarthritis (RF-negative, ANA-negative)
  - polyarthritis (RF-positive)
  - juvenile psoriatic arthritis.
- Involvement is of the joints and soft tissues.

- In the lower limbs the common joints affected are:
  - hip
  - knee
  - ankle
  - subtalar joint.
- There is a wide variety of arthritic foot problems and leg-length differences are not uncommon.
- The management of these foot problems depends on:
  - medical treatment of the arthritis
  - local application of specific measures to the damaged foot
  - prescription of orthoses with appropriate properties for each specific abnormality.

Raynaud 's phenomenon

Raynaud's phenomenon is prominent in scleroderma.

- Digit/s become cold, numb and painful on exposure to cold
- Local hypoxia leads to white digits, cyanosis, reactive rubor
- Temporary loss of sensation.

Treatment

- Keeping the whole body, especially the hands and feet, warm and preventing and protecting the body from cold exposure
- Feet and especially toes should be carefully monitored particularly through the autumn and winter months with prevention and early management of problems being a high priority.

Haemophilia

- Joint swelling and pain often heralds haemarthrosis.
- The correct policy is to encourage the patient to attend hospital at the earliest sign of joint swelling.
- Joint deformity in the foot requires orthotic management to limit damage.

Turner's syndrome

This presents with:

- lymphoedema of the lower limb
- nail dysplasia
- ingrowing toenails due to
  - short, broad feet
  - hyperextension of the great toe
  - involuted toenails
  - oedematous periungual tissues
  - STJ pronation.

Due to the poor lymphatic drainage, girls with Turner's syndrome are at increased risk from cellulitis – so that all cases of infection must be treated diligently and as a matter of urgency.

Down's syndrome (trisomy 21)

- Features of Down's syndrome are evident at birth.
- Physical abnormalities are seen in the face and skull.

- During the first years of life hypotonia and laxity of joints are evident.
- The first and second fingers and/or toes are widely spaced.
- A number of pedal anomalies may be present:
  - hypermobility
  - adducted 1st ray
  - severe pes plano-valgus
  - genu valgum
  - circulatory insufficiency
  - psoriatic arthropathy.

DERMATOLOGICAL CONDITIONS

The most common dermatological conditions seen in childhood are:

- atopic eczema
- dermatitis
- psoriasis, but is more common in the late teens
- juvenile plantar dermatosis
- verrucae
- blisters
- inherited and acquired keratodermas, which may manifest in childhood.

Examination and assessment

Children are constantly being subjected to developmental change by:

- intrinsic factors within the foot
- extrinsic factors within the lower limb and skeleton.

The following examination methodology is employed:

- relaxed, stress-free atmosphere
- observation of gait and posture with footwear
- subjective questioning of child and/or parent
- examination and measurement of feet and footwear
- visual and physical examination of skin, nail, soft-tissue and bony lesions
- examination of range, quality and direction of motion joints
- determine foot type
- biomechanical assessment for forefoot/rearfoot alignment
- assess bare-footed gait and general posture comparing right with left
- compare bare-footed gait and general posture with foot posture and general findings
- make a diagnosis
- produce a management plan
- provide written literature concerning the complaint and treatments.

Physical examination of foot joints

- Ankle
- Subtalar
- Midtarsal
- Metatarsophalangeal
- Interphalangeal.

Joints should be examined for range, quality and direction of motion, comparing right with left.

The range of motion or deformity in joints is recorded using a goniometer for charting and comparison at a later date once treatment has been instigated.

Biomechanical assessment

This can be difficult in the young child. As accurate and thorough an assessment as possible should be carried out.

Observe and assess bare-footed gait and general posture. The following factors should be considered when observing gait and posture in children.

- Head – size, shape, symmetry, facial expression
- Shoulders – level, position
- Spine – kyphosis, lordosis, scoliosis, kyphoscoliosis
- Pelvis – anteroposterior tilting, posteroanterior tilting, lateral tilting, rotation, asymmetry
- Hips – level
- Femur – bowing, internal torsion, external torsion
- Knee – position of patella (inward, forward, outward facing), genu valgum, genu varum, genu recurvatum
- Tibia – internal torsion, external torsion, bowing
- Foot – in-toeing, out-toeing, calcaneal deviation, excessive subtalar joint pronation, forefoot deformity.

Diagnosis

Make a firm diagnosis and record measurements for comparison at a later date. Discuss the findings, treatment options and the potential outcomes with the parents or carers and obtain 'informed consent' to progress with the child's management.

Produce a management plan

Decide whether to treat (there and then or at a later date), monitor or refer.

Written information

Provide the patient/parent with written literature concerning the complaint and associated management.

MANAGEMENT

Many children with foot pathologies are treated in a relatively *ad hoc* fashion with little apparent logic to the management. In order to overcome this, a logical approach is required. Having made a diagnosis, obtained informed consent, and formulated a management plan, all children should be managed similarly utilising a standard convention. This simply involves footwear, exercises and orthoses.

Footwear advice and prescription

Structural foot conditions cannot be managed until suitable footwear and hosiery are obtained. Without the correct footwear the podiatrist is unable to manage the presenting problem.

- Charities provide footwear for children with proven chronic foot disorders if there is a financial burden on the family.
- Children with a disability can be 'over shod' with clumpy, unsuitable and socially unacceptable prescription footwear.
- 'Off the peg' shoes should always be considered.
- The available range of trainers is often suitable unless the deformity is gross or particularly difficult to manage.
- The use of trainers improves the management by providing a suitable vehicle for an orthoses and enhances the child's psychological wellbeing.
- Most hospital orthotic departments supply footwear but this is limited and directed towards the use of rigid ankle/foot orthoses or leg/ankle, foot orthoses.

Passive and active exercises

- Passive exercises stretch tight tissues and mobilise joints and can be complemented by active exercises. Typical examples where this can be employed are:
  - digital deformities
  - shortening of the Achilles tendon
  - active disease within the foot such as juvenile idiopathic arthritis.

Generally, this management is best undertaken by the physiotherapist, but should be incorporated as part of the multidisciplinary approach to care. Hydrotherapy and physical therapies may also be employed at this stage.

Casted foot orthoses

- Consideration is given to the type of device and when to use it.
- In general terms rigid casted orthoses are contraindicated in children undergoing developmental change, although semirigid devices may be considered.
- The majority of cases of STJ pronation relate to compensation for normal physiological change, which should be left alone unless excessive or causing secondary problems.
- When parents are particularly concerned the very young child can be monitored at regular intervals, measurements taken and the parents reassured.
- Orthoses may be used at a later date if required.
- Children affected by systemic disease and neuromuscular conditions must be treated positively. It is best to cast each child individually and not use 'off the shelf' orthoses.
- Parents should be given verbal and written advice regarding the use of orthoses.
- The foot cannot be regarded in isolation. The podiatrist must be satisfied that the primary pathology is intrinsic to the foot. A proximal cause of the condition or of systemic disease indicates referral.

Chapter | **13** |

Sports medicine and injuries

ATHLETIC PROFILE AND HISTORY TAKING

Taking the history of the sporting patient (after Boyd & Bogdan 1997).

Training history

- How many years have you been running?
- How many miles per day do you average?
- How many miles per week do you run?
- What's your longest run during the week or weekend?
- What pace (in minutes per mile/kilometre) do you average in your work-outs?
- Do you do interval training? Track work?
- What type of terrain do you usually run on (dirt, grass, asphalt, concrete, cinder, beach sand, hills, flat, crowned, or track)?
- Do you run on any canted surfaces (on one side of the road, on beaches) or always around a track (in the same direction or opposite directions) clockwise or counterclockwise?
- What time of day do you normally run (a.m., p.m., or mid-day)?

Racing history

- How often do you race?
- Do you compete in 5000 or 10 000 metres or marathons? Do you compete in triathlons?

Running shoe history

- In what brand and model(s) of running shoes do you train and/or race?
- How long have you had your present pair(s) of running shoes?
- Approximately how many miles of wear do you have on your present shoe(s)?

- Do you 'build up' your running shoes to keep the outer soles from wearing out too quickly?
- Where does the most outersole wear occur on your running shoes (inside/outside/back)?
- How do your shoes fit (too long, short, narrow, wide)?
- Do you wear a straight last, curved last or semicurved lasted shoe?
- Do you wear socks when you run? Of what type of material are these made (cotton, acrylic, coolmax)? How many pairs of socks do you wear?
- Are you still wearing the same model shoe more than one time?
- Do any of your pairs of shoes make the problem better or worse?
- Do you wear any orthotics, over-the-counter insoles, special arch supports in your shoes?

Pre/post run activities

- Do you stretch before and/or after your run and for how long?
- What type of stretching do you do (describe it precisely)?
- Do you warm-up/warm-down for your runs and for how long?
- Do you do any muscle-strengthening exercises (weight training)? Describe them.
- Do you participate in any other sports or any other physical activities (cross-training)?
- Do you use a massage therapist?

Injury-related history

- Did you modify your training/racing schedule prior to your injury? Have you increased your mileage significantly in a short period of time?
- Did you run a particularly hard race or have a hard workout immediately prior to your injury?
- Did you switch to another pair of running shoes prior to your injury? How long have you worn them?
- Did you modify your shoe gear prior to your injury?
- Did you adapt to your new orthotics slowly? Over how long a period?
- Was there any direct trauma associated with your injury?
- Did you have another injury or any discomfort in your feet or legs prior to your injury that you tried to train through?
- Have you attempted to compensate your running gait due to any pain or discomfort?
- Have you cut back on your mileage or pace since your injury? Any results?

CHRONIC OR OVERUSE INJURIES

The tissue most commonly affected by over-use injuries is the musculotendinous unit when:

- tension is applied to it quickly
- tension is applied to it obliquely
- the tendon is under tension before loading
- the attached muscle is maximally innervated

Table 13.1 Factors in over-use injuries

EXTRINSIC	INTRINSIC
Training errors	Alignment abnormalities
Time (duration)	Femoral neck anteversion
Distance	Genu valgum
Repetitions (intervals)	Tibial varum
Intensity	Pronation
Hills	Tibial torsion
Surfaces	Limb-length discrepancy
hard (asphalt, concrete)	Muscle weakness
soft (grass, dirt)	
track (cinder, composition)	
canted track	
crowned road	
shoes and equipment	

- the muscle group is stretched by exterior stimuli
- the tendon is weak in comparison with the muscle (Tables 13.1 and 13.2).

FOREFOOT INJURIES

- Skin irritation secondary to mechanical abrasion
- Metatarsalgia
- Capsulitis
- Bursitis
- Sesamoiditis
- Tendinitis
- Neuritis (neuroma)
- Stress fracture
- Nail and toe conditions.

REARFOOT INJURIES

- Pes planus
- Excessive subtalar joint pronation
- Inadequate dorsiflexion (equinus)
- Forefoot varus
- Flexible forefoot valgus
- Functional or structural hallux limitus
- Weakness of the plantar intrinsic musculature
- Chronic traction of the origin of the plantar fascia
- Hypertrophic connective tissue response
- Fibrocartilage proliferation
- Osseous spur formation
- Adventitious bursal development.

Table 13.2 Sports and their injuries

Sport	Knee pain, hip and lower back pain	Tendon rupture and tendinitis	Ankle sprain	Lesser met stress fractures and neuroma	Avulsion fractures	Tinea pedis	HAV/HR and toe problems	Blisters	Shin splints	Nail injuries	Plantar fasciitis	Neuropraxia
Football	X			X	X	X		X	X	X	X	X
Gymnastics			X	X		X		X		X	X	
Basketball		X	X	X				X		X	X	
Bowls	X		X								X	
Tennis	X	X	X	X	X			X		X	X	
Golf	X		X				X					
N American Football	X	X	X	X	X	X	X					X
Rugby	X	X	X	X	X	X	X					X
Aerobics		X		X		X	X				X	
Dance	X	X	X	X	X	X	X	X	X	X	X	
Running	X	X	X	X	X	X	X	X	X	X	X	
Baseball	X	X	X	X		X	X	X		X	X	
Skiing	X	X		X			X	X		X	X	

LEG INJURIES

- Tibial fasciitis is an overuse inflammatory condition localised to the posteromedial crest of the tibia, with occasional involvement to the anterior crest of the tibia.
- This condition has been commonly referred to as posterior and anterior shin splints.

Treatment

- The acute phase is directed towards decreasing pain and inflammation.
- The rehabilitation phase is focused on decreasing the pain and swelling even further while attempting to decrease or prevent the formation of scar tissue, strengthening the deep fascia–bone interface, while maintaining flexibility of surrounding soft-tissue structures. Deep compartment muscle exercise can help to strengthen the deep facial–bone interface while reducing the tension force to the deep facial insertion.
- The functional phase is designed to functionally strengthen the fascial–bone interface and to further prevent the tibia from excessive tension forces.
- The return-to-activity phase is aimed at returning the athlete to his or her desired sport and level of participation.

STRESS FRACTURE OF THE TIBIA AND FIBULA (FATIGUE FRACTURES)

- Caused by muscle fatigue, creating a loss in shock absorption and allowing excessive forces to be transmitted to the underlying bone or repeated muscular forces acting upon the bone.
- Approximately half of all stress fractures in athletes occur in the shaft of the tibia.
- In ballet dancers the middle third of the tibia is commonly involved
- In runners the area most frequently seen is the middle and distal thirds of the tibial shaft.
- Stress fractures may also occur at the medial malleolus due to distance running or basketball or American football.
- Stress fractures of the fibula generally occur in the lower third.
- Stress fractures are also seen in the proximal third of the fibula.
- The more serious anterior midshaft tibia stress fracture may become a complete fracture.

Treatments

- Rest for at least 6–8 weeks
- Longer rest period if necessary to allow for adequate bone healing and to prevent further injury
- A slow, progressive return to full-impact activity is advised, with periods of rest.

ACUTE AND CHRONIC COMPARTMENT SYNDROME

- Compartment syndrome is caused by an increase in tissue pressure to a critical level resulting in a compromise in tissue perfusion.

195

- There are four requisites necessary before the diagnosis of compartment syndrome can be made:
  - a limiting anatomical envelope
  - an increase in tissue pressure
  - compromised circulation
  - neuromuscular dysfunction
- Management is as for shin splints.

MUSCLE CRAMPS

- Pain, a tightening of the muscle group, or both, usually due to muscle fatigue, and the accumulation of metabolites during strenuous exercise.

PATELLOFEMORAL PROBLEMS IN RUNNERS

- Patellofemoral joint pain is one of the most common stress-related injuries experienced and is often called 'Runner's knee syndrome'.
- It is a mild lateral subluxation of the patella not to be mistaken for the chondromalacia patellae disorder.
- Runner's knee syndrome develops as a result of poor running mechanics, malalignment problems, increased 'Q' angle, tibial varum, internal tibial torsion, weakened quadriceps muscle group, hard running surfaces and faulty shoes.
- Women, due to their increased 'Q' angle secondary to an anatomically wider pelvis, are at greater risk for suffering from this disorder.
- Prescription orthoses can help to re-align the foot, thus reducing the 'Q' angle.

CHONDROMALACIA PATELLAE

- Malalignment with recurrent subluxation of the patella is probably one of the most common causes for chondromalacia.
- In cases where recurrent subluxation of the patella occurs, there will be damage to the patellar articular cartilage.
- Caused by a combination of factors that push the patella out of its groove on the femur such as weakness of the vastus medialis muscle; an increased 'Q' angle; malalignment of the lower limb, creating excessive foot pronation, leading to increased tibial torsion, and increased stress upon the knee.
- It is a degenerative process on the retropatellar surface. It has been classified in four stages:
  - Stage I represents a softening or degeneration of the articular cartilage.
  - Stage II reveals a cleaving of the articular cartilage.
  - Stage III shows cleaving and fronding of the articular cartilage.
  - Stage IV is wearing away of the articular cartilage to subchondral bone.

Differential diagnoses

- Eliminate chronic synovitis, meniscal lesions, fat pad syndrome, pre-patellar bursitis, retropatellar bursitis, infrapatellar tendon tendinitis, medial synovial plica syndrome, pes anserinus bursitis and sprain of the retinaculum.

Treatment

- Conservative, consisting of salicylates, non-steroidal anti-inflammatory drugs (NSAIDs), patellar stabilising devices, icing, ultrasound, nerve stimulation, massage, changing running programme and running surfaces:
  - quadriceps exercises and iliotibial band stretching
  - re-alignment of the mal-tracking patella with orthotic therapy
  - surgical intervention to achieve a proximal realignment
  - arthroscopic local debridement of the articular lesion is helpful if confined to one facet or if the chondromalacia is grade II or III.

Iliotibial band friction syndrome (ITBFS)

- This overuse injury affects marathon runners, ultra-runners and cyclists.
- It is an overuse injury caused by excessive friction between the iliotibial band (ITB) as it passes over the lateral femoral excrescence.
- Pain may extend along the course of the iliotibial band, and may radiate proximally or distally. Soft-tissue swelling may be present, and there may be palpable crepitus.
- A test performed by the clinician fully extending flexing the knee. It is this sliding over the femoral excrescence that reproduces the pain.

Treatment

- For the early stages of the condition include adequate stretching and proper warm-up, with heat or topical rub before the run, followed by additional stretching and ice massage afterwards.

POPLITEUS TENDINITIS

- This is a common overuse injury that is seen in downhill runners and skiers, and those with excessive pronation.
- Physical examination reveals localised tenderness overlying the tendinous origin and along the lateral femoral condyle.
- Treatment includes NSAIDs and restricting all downhill running, application of ice for acute symptoms.
- Alleviating stress to the popliteus is important by changing the side of the road or direction on the banked track, and by running uphill – not downhill.

HAMSTRING TENDINITIS

- Injury to the hamstring can occur at any particular site along its course.
- The hamstring will appear to be 'tight'.
- Swelling, ecchymosis and/or haematoma formation will be present.
- Pain will be elicited at the site of the injury, most commonly at the midthigh, or the ischial tuberosity.

- Muscle strengthening and flexibility exercises are essential to prevent recurrent injury.

LEG-LENGTH DISCREPANCY

- A leg length shortage can be either anatomical or physiological.
- The leg-length difference is seen in both neutral calcaneal stance position and relaxed calcaneal stance position.
- Functional leg-length discrepancy may occur in sports where an overdevelopment of one limb produces a significant difference.
- Unilateral conditions such as these include iliotibial band syndrome, unilateral patellofemoral joint syndrome or chondromalacia, unilateral shin splints, unilateral posterior tibial tendinitis or Achilles tendinitis.
- Biomechanical evaluation should include a measurement of both limbs.
- The measurement is taken from the anterior superior iliac spine to the medial malleolus.
- The femoral component should be measured at the joint line of the femur and the tibia.
- It is common for compensations of leg length to be seen in the feet.
- The shorter side will supinate and maintain weight bearing on the outside of the foot while attempting to lengthen the limb.
- It can also function in an equinus position to prevent shortening of the limb.
- The opposite will take place on the long limb side where the foot will pronate more than normally to shorten the limb.
- This will be seen by the excessive medial shoe wear.

Chapter | **14** |

Clinical therapeutics

THE THERAPEUTIC MANAGEMENT OF SUPERFICIAL LESIONS

Operating

- Quick relief of pain related to skin and nail pathologies by skilful painless operating, good skin tension, optimum reduction of pathological tissue, avoidance of haemorrhage, protective padding and strapping. Electrosurgery can also produce good results with intractable lesions in carefully selected patients.

Medicaments

- The majority of preparations used in podiatry are topical applications with specific function, as in chemical caustics, antifungal agents and antiseptics, but generally they are of palliative effect.
- Long-term use of medicaments should be avoided as some agents may cause contact dermatitis.
- Peripheral neuropathy, vascular insufficiency, impaired immune response or the effects of long-term steroid therapy may make the application of caustics cause breakdown of tissue.

Dressings

- Dressings protect from friction, pressure and infection or are sterile and used on areas where the epidermis has been breached.

Padding and strapping

- In foot problems, biomechanical in origin, mechanical therapy has a vital role in correcting function in short-term treatment with adhesive or replaceable padding, or in long-term management by orthoses, footwear advice, modification to footwear or specialised shoes. Combinations of clinical padding and orthoses are also used in management of biomechanical disorders, and silicone and thermoplastic materials are used as a medium or long-term measure

- Adhesive padding protects by: correction, deflection and cushioning, removing tensile or shearing stresses from the epidermis.

COMMON SITES OF SOFT-TISSUE LESIONS

Pathological callous

- Pathological callous, 1st metatarsal head, 5th metatarsal head, 1st and 5th metatarsal head, 2nd, 3rd and 4th metatarsal heads, medial aspect of 1st metatarsal head, lateral aspect of 5th metatarsal head.

Heloma durum

- Heloma durum of the digits – dorsal aspect and apices of the lesser toes, nail sulci associated with pressure from the nail plate, lateral edge of the nail and particularly the 5th toe
- Heloma durum (hard corns) on the plantar metatarsal area associated with common structural deformities pes cavus (under the 1st and 5th metatarsal heads), hallux limitus/rigidus (under the 2nd or 5th metatarsal heads and interphalangeal joint (IPJ) of the hallux), hallux abductovalgus (under the 2nd and 3rd metatarsal heads).

Interdigital heloma

- Interdigital heloma – compression between opposing joints, abnormal digital alignment exacerbated by hypermobility of the feet and excessive pronation, constriction of the toes from footwear, biomechanical problem in the rearfoot, such as a rearfoot varus, hyperhidrosis.

Vascular and neurovascular heloma

- Vascular and neurovascular heloma have vascular and neural elements. Operating is extremely painful, reduction may be incomplete, because of multiple small nuclei, use of Local Anaesthesia or progressive electrosurgery may be required, difficult to eradicate. Repeated applications of 50% silver nitrate solution may be effective. Commonly over plantar aspect of the metatarsal head, areas under excessive pressure.

Heloma miliare (seed corns)

- Associated with anhidrosis and commonly occur on any area of the plantar surface of the feet, medial longitudinal arch and heel. Not associated with pressure.

CASE RECORDS

These are of inestimable value in refuting allegations of malpractice and are the main weapon in the defence of such allegations. They should be accurate, succinct but detailed; contain a current detailed medical, surgical and pharmacological history; conform to a set standard; be legible; be coherent and understandable; be a complete record of treatment; use accepted abbreviations; be completed immediately following treatment; indicate informed consent; record advice given to patient and be maintained in a safe and secure place.

SHORT-TERM PADDING THERAPY (SEE ALSO WEBSITE)

Digital padding for the lesser toes

- Padding should protect, re-distribute pressure, correct function and act as a vehicle for medicaments. In imbalance between the extensor and flexor muscles use combined dorsoplantar splints.

Plantar metatarsal padding

- Plantar padding is used to correct, re-distribute excessive load, protect by cushioning and reduce friction.
- A plantar metatarsal pad is shaped to cover the heads and approximately two-thirds of the shafts of the middle three metatarsals, dorsiflexing them with the full thickness of the pad under the metatarsal heads to realign them and deflection away from the 1st and 5th metatarsal heads relieving symptoms. Clawed or retracted toes need to be corrected with digital dorsoplantar splints.
- Adaptations include single-wing pads (SW/PMP), double wing pads (DW/PMP) and 'U' section cut outs (U/PMP). Fig 14.1
- Metatarsal bars are designed to realign the metatarsophalangeal joints (MTPJs), increase toe function and deflect some pressure from the metatarsal heads on to the metatarsal shafts, and are contoured to the metatarsal formula extending two-thirds along the metatarsal shafts.
- Shaft pads may be used to any metatarsal, although the most common is to the first. Long-shaft pads are used almost exclusively to the 1st metatarsal and extend to the interphalangeal joint (IPJ) to increase the weight bearing

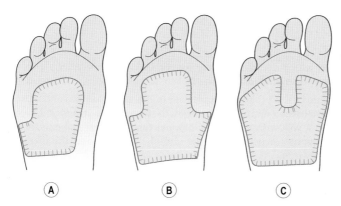

Figure 14.1 Plantar metatarsal padding. (A) Single-wing plantar metatarsal pad (PMP) to the 5th metatarsal head. (B) Double-wing PMP to the 1st and 5th metatarsal heads. (C) 'U' shaped PMP.

through the metatarsal head, limit motion at the MTPJ and deflect pressure away from the IPJ in hallux limitus/rigidus. Short-shaft pads stop distal to the metatarsal heads and are designed to increase the load to a particular metatarsal and realign the MTPJ.

THE TREATMENT OF VERRUCA PEDIS

- The principal measures are chemical cautery, cryotherapy, curettage, electrosurgery, interactive dressings, astringents and homeopathic remedies.
- Considerations prior to treatment: site, number and size, skin texture, circulation, neuropathy, availability of patient, age and previous treatments.

Chemical cautery

Any padding leaves the tissues macerated, making hygiene problematical. It should also be noted that the rate of penetration of the acid cannot be predicted easily. However, chemical treatment can guarantee rapid results, although all forms of treatment will cause a degree of discomfort or pain and inconvenience. Hyperhidrosis is a contraindication:

- salicylic acid ointments, pastes, solutions and collodion from 20 to 75%. In solution or a collodion base, it is easily confined and limited to the area of the verruca and produces a mild localised action.
- monochloroacetic acid – rarely used due to a high incidence of tissue breakdown and scarring.
- trichloroacetic acid – is slow and controlled if used at its usual concentration of 10%.

Single-treatment techniques

- Cryotherapy, using liquid nitrogen or nitrous oxide
- Electrosurgery, using coagulation, desiccation or fulguration, by 'hot-wire' cautery or with electrosurgical units
- Curettage.

These treatments do not entail frequent return visits. Padding is, usually, only necessary to relieve pressure after treatment if the verruca is on a weight-bearing area.

Cryotherapy

- Nitrous oxide, with a release of temperature of 88.5°C
- Liquid nitrogen operating temperature of 196°C.

With both methods use a probe-size equivalent to that of the verruca and a conducting medium such as a macrogol jelly. Begin the freeze and watch for the halo, which is seen as a yellowish white ring. Normal time of freeze is between 30 seconds and 2 minutes depending on the size of the lesion and the method chosen.

Liquid nitrogen requires less freezing time than nitrous oxide. Allow the tissues to thaw at normal room temperature. When normal colour returns a repeat freeze should be carried out.

Silver nitrate may be applied over the verruca if desired to harden the superficial tissues and prevent rupture of the blister. Apply a protective dressing to the area, which usually requires padding on weight-bearing surfaces. The patient should be seen again in 1 week to assess the effectiveness of the treatment. At this stage a blister should have formed around the entire lesion. The lesion may be cut out at this stage and the resultant ulcer treated with an appropriate broad-spectrum antiseptic until healing is complete. Alternatively the patient may be left for up to 6 weeks when the blister will have resolved and the dead verruca tissue removed with a scalpel.

Electrosurgery

Patient selection

- Local infiltration or nerve blockade anaesthesia is required before treatment. Desiccation of a corn or verruca is not recommended where healing is severely compromised and should not be carried out if the patient has a metal implant between the lesion to be treated and the site of the dispersal plate. There is potential risk of interference with pacemakers.

Procedures

- *Cutting* – to cut tissue, an undamped or mildly damped current with a very fine emitting electrode is used.
- *Fulguration* – for electrofulguration, a high-voltage damped waveform is used.
- *Desiccation* – an intermittent, damped waveform with a relatively high voltage and low current is used.
- *Coagulation* – it is achieved electrosurgically using a current relatively lower in voltage and higher in amperage than for desiccation. Ball or flat probes are often used in this way to coagulate small blood vessels and stop bleeding. Very precise haemostasis may be obtained by using bipolar forceps. Each blade is connected to the radiosurgical unit so the current passes between the two blades. This may be useful in microsurgery where individual vessels can be coagulated.
- *Electrosurgical treatment of verrucae* – verrucae can be removed by cutting with a loop electrode, or they can be desiccated using the procedure for desiccation of chronic corns.
- *Nail bed ablation* the procedure is facilitated by using a specially designed matrixectomy electrode which is insulated on one side to prevent damage to the overlying eponychium. The tourniquet remains in place following partial or total nail avulsion. The probe is held lightly over the nail bed and activated for 2–4 seconds. The probe is moved and the process is repeated until all areas of the germinal epithelium have been treated. Normally bleeding is not a problem due to the desiccating effect.
- *Procedure for desiccation of heloma durum (hard corn).* A local anaesthetic is administered. Overlying callus or corn is reduced with a scalpel. A suitable probe is selected. The area to be treated is swabbed with sterile saline; repeated throughout the procedure to allow maximum desiccation and prevent superficial charring. Application should be for approximately 2 seconds. Blanching of the tissues should occur. Once the blanching has been achieved, the process is repeated around the lesion periphery with each area of blanching interconnecting. Continue until the whole lesion is desiccated. The blunt edge of a scalpel may be used to work around the periphery of the blanched area to loosen it. Desiccation will have caused separation at the dermo-epidermal junction. Remove all of the desiccated tissue, to reveal the underlying dermis.

INFLAMMATORY CONDITIONS

Perniosis (erythema pernio, chilblains)

Chilblains can be divided into four stages: the *cyanotic* stage, the *hyperaemic* stage, followed by the *congestive* stage and the *ulcerative* or broken chilblain stage. In the hyperaemic stage the application of cold compresses is essential to control the symptoms of this stage. At the congestive stage stimulate the local circulation with rubefacients, vasodilator creams or the application of heat. Heat can be applied via the use of an infrared heat lamp, wax baths or a warm footbath.

TREATMENT OF DISORDERS OF THE SWEAT GLANDS

Hyperhidrosis

- It is important to appraise all footwear worn by the patient and also the demands of their occupation. Various treatment strategies can be adopted ranging from the application of dusting powders, swabbing with an astringent lotion, to the administration of footbaths containing an astringent medicament.
- Crystals of potassium permanganate dissolved in a footbath are effective. When the maceration has ceased, the footbaths should be reduced to twice weekly.
- Footbaths containing 3% formalin may also be used.
- Spirit-based astringent agents can be used if there is excessive maceration in conjunction with the application of dusting powders.
- The patient should be advised to dispense with shoes and socks whenever possible, or to wear sandals, to pay particular attention to foot hygiene and to change hosiery daily and to alternate footwear.

Anhidrosis

- The choice of emollient matters little since the purpose is to prevent moisture loss from the skin. Hydrous lanolin, E45 cream, white soft paraffin, urea-based preparations or proprietary medicaments incorporating lanolin are suitable. The main complication of anhidrosis is the formation of fissures due to the reduction of epidermal elasticity and applied tensile stress commonly found on the borders of the heel, which is associated with callus formation.
- Treatment consists of careful reduction of the callus at the edges of the fissures, treatment with an antiseptic cream and an occlusive dressing for a few days.

TREATMENT OF FUNGAL INFECTIONS

Tinea pedis

- The common causative organisms in the United Kingdom in order of frequency are: *Trichophyton rubrum*, *Trichophyton interdigitale*, *Epidermophyton floccosum*, *Microsporum canis* (cat and dog ringworm), *Trichophyton verrucosum* and *Trichophyton mentagrophytes*.

- General issues regarding treatment should be: identifying the probable source if possible, advice on avoidance, foot hygiene and type of footwear.
- Advice should be given to eliminate barefoot contact with all surfaces, which are liable to be contaminated. Personal foot hygiene should be of the highest standard, the feet should be meticulously dried and the shared use of towels or footwear should be avoided.

Clinical features of tinea pedis

- In its mildest form it may be confused with erythrasma and the symptoms negligible. In the more severe form there is associated inflammation, maceration, fissuring, bleeding, blistering and the possibility of a superimposed bacterial infection.
- Interdigital areas are most commonly affected in the first instance. The appearance can vary from simple scaling of the skin with minimal itching, to macerated raw areas with spread of the infection to the under-surface of the toes or to the dorsum of the foot with blistering and inflammation.
- There may well be a superimposed bacterial infection with Gram-negative bacteria, commonly of the *Pseudomonas* type. Blistering is usually associated with *Trichophyton interdigitale*. The sole of the foot in the area of the medial longitudinal arch may be affected. The skin in this area tends to be dry, flaky and inflamed with associated blistering. Fungal infections can spread to any area of the skin or to the nails.

Treatment

Fungicidal preparations can be applied as creams, ointments, lotions, aerosol sprays and powders, effective if the infection is not widespread or involves nails. Topical therapy with specific antifungal preparations leaves the practitioner and patient a wide choice from which to choose. The following are some of the most commonly used preparations:

- *undecenoic acid* – preparations containing undecenoic acid are Monphytol, Mycota, Phytocil and Tineafax.
- *tolnaftate* – available as Tinaderm and Timoped.
- *the imidazoles* – these are available as Ecostatin and Pevaryl and 2% miconazole (available as Daktarin and Dermonistat).
- *tea tree oil* – (oil from the plant *Melaleuca alternifolia*) is considered to have an antifungal action which may make it useful in the topical treatment of fungal infections.

Tinea unguium (onychomycosis)

Clinical features

Fungal infections of the nails will be seen as thickened and crumbly with a yellowish discoloration and eventually the whole nail plate may be involved. If the use of antifungal agents does not prevail the nail plate may be avulsed with or without phenolisation of the matrix. When the use of local analgesia is contraindicated, medical avulsion may be attempted with the use of 40% urea cream, and thereafter topical antifungal preparations applied as described above.

Treatment

Systemic treatment of onychomycosis is probably the treatment of choice in adults.

Candida

Candida infections can affect both skin and nail; the most common sites in the foot to be affected are the interdigital spaces and the nail. The nail plate itself may become infected in association with paronychia. The nail plate will not become thickened, but onycholysis and destruction of the distal end of the nail plate may result. Most of the superficial *Candida* infections respond to topical applications of the azoles, Terbinafine or Nystatin. For paronychia the treatment should be in solution form to enable it to run into the nail folds, and treatment should be continued for 3–4 months. Oral therapy with terbinafine, itraconazole or ketoconazole is necessary when the nail plate is involved.

PHYSICAL THERAPY

Physical therapy can be defined as the treatment of disease or injury by physical means, such as light, heat, cold water, electricity, massage and exercise. It may be used effectively, in conjunction with padding, tension strapping and an orthotic device, as a management strategy in podiatric practice without the use of pharmacological preparations or invasive treatments.

Heat and cold have been used as methods of treatment for trauma since 400 BC. The local physiological effects of heat and cold help many of the adverse local pathological changes which occur as a result of the tissue damage. The cardinal signs and symptoms of inflammation (rubor, calor, dolor and tumor) may be reduced, healing assisted and rehabilitation time improved. Heat may be applied to the skin by conduction using a hot pack or, conversely, cold through the use of an ice pack. Radiation is where an object when heated emits infrared rays (and possibly also visible and ultraviolet rays), for example, dry heat in the form of infrared lamps.

Heat

When heat is used as a method of treatment it must be remembered that heating of tissues beyond 45°C causes irreversible damage of tissue proteins and death of tissues.

Infrared radiation

This forms part of the electromagnetic spectrum, and cannot be seen. Artificial infrared radiation is generally produced by passing an electrical current through a coiled resistant wire and can be used clinically as either luminous or non-luminous.

The non-luminous generator produces long rays and is absorbed in the tissues of the epidermis. The luminous generator produces shorter rays which penetrate to the dermis and subcutaneous tissues and can cause irritation of the tissues. The application of infrared rays leads to a local rise in temperature with a subsequent increase in the blood supply to the area, relief of pain, muscle relaxation and elimination of waste products.

The lamp should be positioned so that its rays strike the part to be treated at a right angle and at a distance of 45–61 cm (18–24 inches). The surrounding tissues should be covered for protection. Changing the distance of the lamp from the area to be treated, if no control switch is available, can alter the intensity. The duration of treatment should be 15 minutes and may be repeated on a daily basis.

Infrared can be used effectively on chronic musculoskeletal and traumatic conditions such as sprains, strains, plantar fasciitis and arthropathies.

Skin which has had liniment, oil or embrocation cream applied to it recently should not be treated with this form of heat, as this may enhance the heating effect and cause superficial blistering. Acute inflammation, evidence of bleeding, sepsis, other skin conditions or circulatory impairment are also contraindications.

Ultrasound

Thermal effects

When ultrasound travels through tissues a percentage is absorbed, leading to the generation of heat within the tissues. As the waves pass through the different tissues or media of the body (skin, muscle, tendon, etc.) they will be subject to varying refractions and scatter. As a result, the intensity of an ultrasound beam decreases as it penetrates deeper into the tissues, referred to as 'half-value distance'. The half-value depth for soft, irregular connective tissue is approximately 4 mm at 3 MHz, but about 11 mm at 1 MHz. The amount of absorption will depend on the nature of the tissue, the vascularity of the area and the frequency of the ultrasound. Tissues with high protein content will absorb more easily than those with a high fat content.

Non-thermal effects/physical properties

Cavitation

Ultrasound can cause the formation of microsized bubbles or cavities in gas-containing fluids. These bubbles can be either useful or dangerous. Cavitation may be unstable and collapse of the bubbles will occur resulting in an excessive rise in local temperature. This can best be avoided by continually moving the treatment head and by using intensities below 3 watts/cm². Stable cavitation is not dangerous and can have beneficial effects.

Acoustic streaming

This describes the unidirectional movement of a fluid in an ultrasound field. Acoustic streaming can accelerate tissue repair as a result of increased capillary permeability, stimulation of activity of mast cells and fibroblasts and the increased production of growth factors by macrophages.

Standing waves

When an ultrasound wave encounters the interface between tissues with different acoustic abilities, for example bone and muscle, reflection of a percentage of the wave will occur. The reflected wave can interact with oncoming waves to form a standing wave field in which the peaks of intensity of the waves are stationary and are separated by half a wavelength. This causes gas bubbles to collect and cause damage to endothelial cells and tissue in the immediate area. This can be avoided by moving the head of the transducer continuously throughout the treatment.

Method of application

Ultrasound can be applied either directly or indirectly to the area being treated. Direct application is achieved by placing the treatment head in contact with the skin via a coupling gel. It is essential to maintain continuous contact between the whole of the treatment face and the skin to avoid damage to the quartz crystal in the transducer. While maintaining an even pressure the treatment head is moved in a circular or figure-of-eight motion over the surface.

Indirect application

- This is achieved by immersing the area to be treated in a water bath. The water medium acts as the conductor between the tissue and the transducer. This is particularly useful for irregular surfaces such as the dorsal aspect of the foot and the 1st MTPJ.
- The foot should be placed in a non-metallic basin containing water, preferably distilled water to avoid air bubbles but this is not essential. Select dosage and continually move treatment head parallel to the part in a circular motion about a quarter of an inch (about 6 mm) from the skin.
- Ultrasound therapy can also be used in conjunction with topical non-steroidal anti-inflammatory preparations. This method is considered to improve the management of a variety of musculoskeletal conditions and acute sports injuries. It is thought that ultrasound may enhance the penetration of some drugs across the skin by the process of phonophoresis.

Suggested treatment dosages used in podiatry

- Intensity:
  - low for recent and acute conditions – 0.25 to 0.5 Watts/cm^2
  - medium for chronic conditions – 0.8 to 1.0 Watts/cm^2
- Frequency:
  - high frequencies are absorbed more rapidly and, therefore, are more suitable for superficial tissues
  - low frequencies penetrate deeper
- Time:
  - start with a short time, e.g. 3 minutes, which can then be increased in subsequent applications
- Pulsed/continuous mode:
  - continuous – thermal effect (chronic conditions)
  - pulsed – non-thermal effects (acute conditions).

Ultrasound can be beneficial in the treatment of soft-tissue injuries, inflammatory conditions, such as painful hallux limitus, and rheumatic and arthritic conditions, but it is contraindicated when infection is present in the area as there is danger of the infection spreading. Ultrasound should never be used if there is a history of deep venous thrombosis as there may be a risk of embolism.

Cold

Cold has the converse effect of heat resulting in vasoconstriction. This will reduce the metabolic rate of tissues resulting in a lowered demand for oxygen and nutrients, thus reducing the effect of the chemical mediators of inflammation and minimising the inflammatory process.

It is useful in the initial treatment of acute trauma such as sprains, as it will limit the initial inflammatory response limiting tissue swelling and pain. However, it should be avoided in patients who are elderly or who have peripheral vascular disease, Raynaud's disease, sensitivity to cold, peripheral neuropathy or cardio-vascular disease.

Cryotherapy

This is the therapeutic application of cold and it can be used in podiatric practice in a variety of circumstances from the application of an ice pack for an acute traumatic incident to the use of freezing techniques for the destruction of skin lesions such as verrucae (see above). Cold can be a very effective treatment in the acute stages of an inflammatory response. It can be applied as follows:

- crushed ice or ice cube packs/frozen peas in towels or cloths
- frozen gel packs
- cold or cooling sprays
- iced water
- cryogenic equipment.

Ice packs

- Placed onto the affected area for approximately 10–15 minutes between layers of a dampened towel. Unopened packets of frozen peas or sweet corn are also useful if quantities of crushed ice are not available.

Gel packs

- These are available in different shapes and sizes and are particularly useful when dealing with sports injuries as they have the benefit of their being able to be used either hot or cold. The gel does not go solid when frozen so it can be easily moulded to the affected area. They can be stored in the freezer compartment of a refrigerator.

Cold sprays

- These are most effective in the initial stages of a traumatic injury. They are applied to the area in short applications of 5–10 seconds over a 2–3-minute period. The skin is cooled quickly by the evaporation of the spray.

Footbaths

- Footbaths can be used effectively in podiatry practice as an alternative treatment regimen as more than one surface can be treated at a time – especially useful for hands and feet.
- Immersion of the foot in a bath containing cold water with ice added for 5–10 minutes for acute traumatic injury. Care must be taken when using this treatment regimen as the patient can experience extreme pain.

Contrast footbaths

This is where the foot is alternately placed in a footbath of warm water and cold water. The foot should be initially placed in the warm water (45–48°C) for 10 minutes and then plunged into the cold for 1 minute. It is then placed back in the warm for 2 minutes and then cold for 1 minute. Continue this for 20 minutes and finish with the cold.

Warm-water footbaths

These are useful for providing diffuse local heat and can also be used as a vehicle for various medicaments. The water should be maintained at a constant temperature of 45°C. It may be necessary on a few occasions to give the patient a footbath for general hygiene purposes. In these cases a suitable detergent such as Hibiscrub (4% w/v chlorhexidine) could be added to the water. Sodium bicarbonate or sodium chloride may be added to the water as antidote in the event of an adverse reaction to strong acids.

A hypertonic footbath

This may be used when sepsis is present to facilitate the drainage of pus from the wound by osmosis. One hundred grams of either magnesium sulphate or sodium chloride should be dissolved in 5 litres of water. The temperature should be kept constant at 46°C for 10–15 minutes.

209

Antiseptic astringent footbaths

These baths containing potassium permanganate crystals or Permitabs are useful in the treatment of hyperhidrosis or bromidrosis, and are used once or twice daily for 10–15 minutes depending on the severity of the condition. A few crystals of potassium permanganate, sufficient to turn the water pale pink, or one Permitab are dissolved in a basin of water at 38°C.

Footbaths are contraindicated if the patient has impaired arterial supply, neuropathy or thin friable skin. Footbaths should also be avoided if there is a break in the skin, fungal infection or verruca.

Lasers

Lasers for therapeutic reasons such as pain reduction, tissue healing and verrucae pedis are becoming increasingly popular today. The word LASER is an acronym for:

- light
- amplification by
- stimulated
- emission of
- radiation.

Properties of laser light

A combination of properties makes laser light unique, allowing for the treatment of specific conditions. Some of the important features within laser light are:

- monochromatic: narrow band width, single wavelength of light
- coherent: waves of light move in step and constant over time
- collimated: beams of light are parallel (small spot size over relatively large distance).

Treatment with laser therapy produces biochemical and photological effects within the cells and tissues. The radiation which is emitted is athermic. All of these stimulatory effects are known as biomodulation. Local metabolic changes occur such as increased inflammatory response, effects on the immune system and increased formation of capillaries, as well as a number of other effects, which are of therapeutic value. The biomodulation effects have been shown to be dose-dependent.

Treatment technique

The painful area should be pinpointed each time and the target area should be in its optimum position to receive treatment. The laser probe should be held at 90° to the skin. Different treatment techniques should be used depending on the area being treated. The probe should be in contact with the skin; the distance between the probe and treatment area should be minimal to prevent divergence of the beam and, therefore, effective treatments.

Contraindications:

- direct treatment of the eye (unless by qualified personnel within the area)
- treatment over pregnant uterus
- presence of active neoplasm
- area of haemorrhage
- transplants.

Cautions:

- treatment over the epiphyseal lines of the bones of children
- irradiation of gonads
- photosensitive tissue.

Indications for use:

- trigger points and acupuncture points
- bone repair
- verrucae pedis
- pain relief (acute and chronic)
- myofascial pain and dysfunction
- rheumatoid arthritis
- osteoarthritis
- neuralgias
- soft-tissue and overuse injuries
- wounds
- bed sores
- burns
- scar tissue.

The patient may experience an increase in pain flare up due to the cellular changes taking place, as the pain is made acute when the healing process starts. It is important that the patient be informed of this before treatment commences so that they are aware of what to expect.

The treatment should be adapted to the patient's needs and its effect should be reviewed at each treatment session and adapted accordingly. This can be included as part of a treatment plan; for example, in wound healing, regular debridement, padding and dressing will be done.

Non-steroidal anti-inflammatory drugs (NSAIDs) and steroids inhibit the effect of laser therapy; therefore, special consideration should be taken when the therapeutic effect is reviewed.

Laser promotes wound healing by having an increased cellular effect resulting in a faster rate of wound healing; however, wounds treated by laser may initially appear to deteriorate, and there may be an increase in the amount of discharge produced, so the patient must be informed of this prior to treatment.

Magnetopulse

Magnetopulse therapy aims to influence the electrical activity across the group of cells being treated to stimulate a faster natural healing rate. Magnetopulse therapy has two basic functions:

- first, to suppress the symptoms of an injury or illness, such as inflammation with associated pain
- second, to treat the cause of the same condition by increased blood flow to the injured area.

It can be used in podiatric practice in the treatment of sports injuries, osteoarthritis and rheumatoid arthritis.

Magnetopulse is contraindicated for pregnant patients and for those with tuberculosis or a viral illness; it should not be used (i) in juvenile diabetes, (ii) if there is a history of thrombosis, (iii) if the patient is susceptible to haemorrhage, or (iv) if the patient has a pacemaker.

When using magnetopulse the clinician must remove all watches and ensure that the machine is kept away from all other electronic equipment such as computers.

For more information see
Neale's Disorders of the Foot 8E *pages 425–426*

Non-thermal electrotherapy

Faradism

Faradism involves the use of a low-frequency current, 50–100 Hz, producing a tetanic muscle contraction, which would be very uncomfortable, so the current is surged to produce an alternative contraction and relaxation of the muscles similar to the normal muscle contraction of muscles with a normal nerve supply. It is used to facilitate muscle contraction when the patient finds it difficult to produce effective muscle action.

Technique

The technique for this is described in Chapter 16 of the 8th edition of *Neale's Disorders of the Foot*.

For more information see
Neale's Disorders of the Foot 8E *pages 426–427*

Interferential

Interferential is where two medium-frequency alternating currents of differing frequencies from 400 Hz to 4250 Hz are applied to the body. Where they cross, they 'interfere' with each other and set up a beat frequency. This low-frequency current can be varied between 0 and 250 Hz to produce different physiological effects. There may be an effect on the pain gate by the short-duration pulses at 80 Hz. Endorphin release can be activated by 2.5 or 130 Hz. The pumping action on the blood vessels speeds up the metabolic rate and the removal of metabolites (0–100 Hz or 0–250 Hz). There will be contraction of muscle between 0 and 100 Hz. This is deeper in the tissues than is the case with faradism, although 0–50 Hz can be effective for the more superficial layers, but the patient cannot contract with it. The pumping action is very effective for the absorption of exudate.

The technique for this is described in Chapter 16 of the 8th edition of *Neale's Disorders of the Foot*.

For more information see
Neale's Disorders of the Foot 8E *page 427*

ACUTE AND CHRONIC INFLAMMATORY CONDITIONS

Acute and chronic inflammatory conditions arising from trauma and/or bursitis may require two methods of treatment complementing each other. The first aims to reduce and control inflammation and swelling by the application of cold when the inflammation is in the acute stage achieved by cold compresses or ice packs.

When the inflammation is chronic, and congestion of the area is evident, mild heat in the form of ultrasound is recommended. Therapeutic laser or magnetopulse therapy are invaluable to hasten the healing process. A major advantage of magnetopulse is that the padding and strapping need not be removed during treatment. The second method is to support and rest the affected part by the use of padding and strapping. Padding can be applied directly to the foot or inserted into the patient's footwear as a transitional stage pending the manufacture and fitting of orthoses. Although orthotic therapy is essential in the longer term, immediate relief or reduction of pain is primarily achieved by padding and strapping.

Tension strappings

- Figure-of-eight strapping for the foot and ankle as shown in Fig 14.2 is used for various conditions:
  - to support a sprained or weak ankle, either inversion or eversion sprains
  - to support a strained foot
  - to limit painful movement in the subtalar and midtarsal joints
  - to relieve tensile stress on the plantar fascia and its calcaneal attachment.

Medial support

Medial support is required, with or without the addition of valgus padding or 'D' pads, in cases of sprain of the deltoid ligament, acute or chronic foot strain and plantar fasciitis. Conversely, it may be applied in such a way as to support the structures on the lateral side of the foot and ankle. Lateral support is required, with or without a tarsal platform or 'filler pad', in cases of sprain of the external lateral ligaments of the ankle, and in some cases of pes cavus with associated postural instability. It may also be applied to hold the foot in a neutral position and to reduce tensile stress on the plantar aspect of the foot, and limit the motions in all directions. This is indicated in arthritis of the tarsal region.

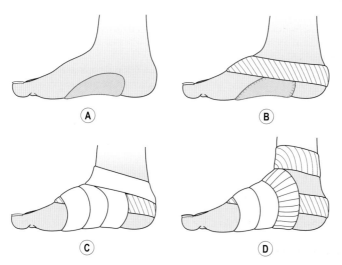

Figure 14.2 Figure-of-eight strapping for the foot and ankle. (A) Valgus or 'D' pad. (B) Non-stretch strapping applied first to invert the heel. (C) Figure-of-eight elastic strapping. (D) Second application of non-stretch reinforcing strapping.

The strapping of choice is a 5 cm (2 inches) or 6.25 cm (2½ inches) elastic adhesive bandage. This is preferable to non-stretch strapping, particularly where oedema is present, as it is less constricting. If hyperhidrosis is present or the patient is allergic to this material it may be applied over a soft cotton bandage. On the dorsum of the foot in order to prevent the plaster sticking to hair, cotton wool can be dragged across the sticky surface of the strapping to that area only.

The technique for the application of *medial support, lateral support and neutral support* is described in detail in Chapter 16 of the 8th edition of *Neale's Disorders of the Foot*.

For more information see
Neale's Disorders of the Foot 8E *pages 427–428*

Valgus padding

This has two separate elements, a plantar cushion and a medial flange. The plantar cushion fills the concavity of the longitudinal arch supporting the joints and the muscular and ligamentous attachments. It is essentially palliative in function. The medial flange extends towards, and if necessary over, the prominences of the sustentaculum tali and the tuberosity of the navicular. Its function is to encourage some degree of inversion of the foot and thereby some correction of abnormal pronation. This is achieved by the pressure of the padding against the firm counter of the shoe.

Applications

- As part of a 'figure-of-eight' strapping for footstrain, a thin felt pad having both elements is usually required Fig 14.2A
- As a temporary palliative orthosis or shoe insert, the plantar element alone may be adequate to control symptoms
- As a permanent feature of an accommodative insole for pes plano-valgus, both elements are usually required in combination with medial heel wedging. The shape, texture and density of the materials used must be varied to suit the needs of each case and will depend on whether the objective is correction or palliation
- In metatarsalgia and in hallux rigidus, with the addition of metatarsal padding or a shaft pad respectively. It is contraindicated in the presence of occlusive arterial disease as it may compress and occlude the plantar arteries and exacerbate or initiate the symptoms of intermittent claudication in the foot nor should it be used alone and continuously as a form of so-called 'arch support'.

Tarsal platform ('filler pad')

This is a short-term measure used as a component of orthoses or as an insert in footwear. Its main function is to bring the lateral border of a highly arched foot into firm contact with the waist of the shoe and tends to evert the foot. It is useful where there is peroneal strain.

Applications

- In *pes cavus*, to re-distribute weight from the heel and metatarsal heads
- In *persistent ankle sprain*, to stabilise the foot by obviating forced inversion

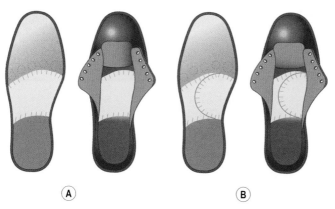

(A)   (B)

Figure 14.3 Tarsal cradle (combination of platform and valgus or 'D' pad).

- In *painful heel*, in conjunction with a heel cushion. The combination is more effective than heel cushioning alone and is indicated in all such cases regardless of the height of the longitudinal arch
- In *metatarsalgia* and plantar lesions in conjunction with suitably shaped metatarsal padding
- In *tarsal arthritis* in conjunction with valgus padding to form a tarsal cradle.

Tarsal cradle

This (Fig 14.3) is a combination of a tarsal platform with a valgus support superimposed. It provides support for both medial and lateral borders of the foot and restrains the movements of inversion and eversion. Its main use is in tarsal arthritis when it may be used to augment the effect of a neutral 'figure-of-eight' strapping. Like the tarsal platform it is not applied to the foot but is used as a component of an insole or as an insert in the footwear. It is also important in restraining hypermobility and elongation of the foot in cases of abnormal pronation associated with calcaniocuboid subluxation.

Padding and strapping for hallux abductovalgus

- It is beneficial to use adhesive padding as a temporary measure prior to the manufacture of orthoses.
- On a younger patient with incipient hallux abductovalgus (HAV) it lessens the deviation of the hallux and thereby relieves the strain on the periarticular tissues and protects the medial eminence from shoe pressure.
- In an established case of HAV where correction is impossible, podiatric management consists of protection of the medial eminence by means of a felt crescent or oval cavity pad.
- If the degree of HAV deformity is greater than the width of the footwear, modifications in the form of balloon patches are essential to relieve pressure from the area.
- The strapping of choice is adhesive stockinette, or similar, which has one-way stretch only cut into a flask or 'butterfly' shape, the anterior ends are first adhered to the hallux and secured there by a narrow strapping.
- The main part of the stockinette is then drawn back over the joint with sufficient tension to correct the line of the hallux to the extent required.
- The 'wings' are then stretched laterally across the dorsal and plantar surfaces of the metatarsal and adhered, covering any padding which has been applied to the joint. Fig 14.4

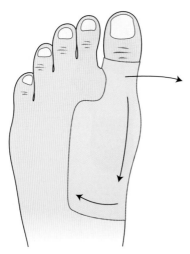

Figure 14.4 Flask strapping to realign hallux abductus. The strapping is adhered around the hallux, below the interphalangeal joint; the hallux is passively moved from its abducted position, then the strapping is applied with sufficient tension over the prominence and the medial side of the foot before being stretched laterally.

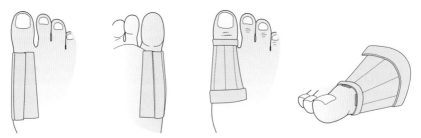

Figure 14.5 Fan strapping for hallux limitus. May be used alone as illustrated or used in conjunction with a shaft pad.

Padding and strapping for hallux limitus/rigidus

- Normally padding or strapping to reduce movement and relieve pressure on the 1st MTPJ on weight bearing is sufficient.
- A single-wing metatarsal pad is often the most readily tolerated padding as it relieves the load on the painful joint, facilitates the inverted position of the foot which is adopted in such cases, and thus helps to minimise dorsiflexion at the joint.
- Pain at the 1st MTPJ which is produced on movement can be alleviated by means of a long shaft pad applied with rigid 'fan' strapping.
- If there is insufficient room within the shoe then the 'fan' strapping may be applied alone. This strapping utilises rigid adhesive strapping of 2.5 cm (1 inch) width (Fig 14.5). With the 1st MTPJ held in the neutral position the strapping is applied from a point just proximal to the interphalangeal joint of the great toe to the base of the 1st metatarsal. The methodology is described in Chapter 16 of the 8th edition of *Neale's Disorders of the Foot*.

··
: **For more information see**
: **Neale's Disorders of the Foot 8E** *pages 430–431*
··

- When strapping is contraindicated the joint can be immobilised by the temporary use of a leatherboard template with a shaft adhered to its undersurface made from either a thin rigid polythene material or other rigid material.

Plantar digital neuritis

- A plantar metatarsal pad with a 'U' to the painful area is most often effective when applied with a full metatarsal strapping.
- Alternatively a short shaft pad, 2–4 PMP or a metatarsal bar may be used.

Plantar fasciitis

- The use of figure-of-eight strapping to invert the calcaneus, either alone or in conjunction with a tarsal platform, is helpful.
- When the pain is primarily along the medial longitudinal arch and there is limited sign of abnormal pronation the use of *bow* strapping is effective in obtaining short-term relief (Fig 14.6). Rigid strapping is used for this purpose in two widths: 2.5 cm (1 inch) for the bands running from the metatarsal head to the heel, and 3.75 cm (1½ inches) for the strapping across the plantar from the lateral to the medial sides of the foot.
- The methodology is described in Chapter 16 of the 8th edition of *Neale's Disorders of the Foot*.

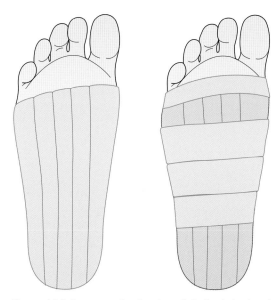

Figure 14.6 Bow strapping for the relief of pain in the plantar fascia.

> **For more information see**
> **Neale's Disorders of the Foot 8E** *page 432*

March fracture

- Relief from pain on weight bearing can be achieved in the short term and sometimes for the duration of the treatment by means of a 7-mm plantar metatarsal pad with a deep 'U' cut out over the affected metatarsal and held in place by a strapping.

Freiberg's infraction

- In the short term the padding of choice is a plantar metatarsal pad with a 'U' to the affected metatarsal head combined with a metatarsal bar to remove as much pressure as possible on weight bearing.

Chapter | **15** |

Orthoses

Podiatrists commonly use a variety of clinical therapies. However, one therapeutic technique has become particularly associated with the profession and that is orthoses.

The use of orthoses is based on the premise that most foot problems have some mechanical factor involved in their aetiology/symptomatology. The basic treatment philosophy for pain or pathology resulting from abnormal foot mechanics is that of control by mechanical means. This may be achieved by either accommodating deformity or altering structure through:

- the use of silicone orthodigita
- surgical intervention to realign bones or to improve soft tissue function
- the use of an orthosis to optimise the function of the foot and lower limb
- the use of combined surgical and orthotic management.

  Post-operative function may be further enhanced with physiotherapy.
  Orthoses may be:

- corrective – realigning anatomical components
- functionally corrective – influence function to modify stress on pathological tissues
- accommodative – primarily accommodate and protect deformities without correcting them.

MATERIALS

Where correction is possible, even if only partial, the corrective element should take precedence over the protective element and this consideration determines the choice of materials.

Thermoplastic materials

The rigidity of materials used in the manufacture of functional orthoses depends on a number of factors:

Temperature

- Higher thermoforming temperature – stronger material
- Lower thermoforming temperature – more likely to deform under load.

Thickness

- Thicker – more rigid
- Thinner – more easily deformable under load.

Carbon fibre composite materials now offer the practitioner a light, thin and flexible alternative. However, they are difficult to use, requiring a higher forming temperature and a shorter working time. Carbon fibre orthoses tend also to be more expensive.

Design

Orthoses should be:

- tolerable to wear
- optimally effective in their therapeutic design.

Manner of application

Orthoses may be:

- worn on the foot, e.g. silicone orthodigita, plantar pads with metatarsal bands
- worn within footwear, e.g. insoles.

Footwear requirements

Orthoses and footwear must be considered together if the optimal outcome is to be achieved. The footwear must:

- be of the correct size and shape
- have adequate internal volume in the right places
- be correctly balanced both mediolaterally and anteroposteriorly
- be modified to ensure the above points.

Heel height

Heel height is of critical importance when fitting a functional orthosis. If heel height is such that the normal relationship between the forefoot and rearfoot is disturbed, then the shoe is totally unsuited to wear with the orthosis.

Semi-bespoke footwear

Stock orthopaedic shoes are now available providing the opportunity to provide a comprehensive orthosis and shoe regimen for many pathologies and an insole system that can be removed to facilitate the fitting of prescribed orthoses.

PRINCIPLES OF MANAGEMENT

These should encompass:

- a management plan devised in consultation with the patient
- the rationale for orthosis therapy
- the concept that other treatments are likely to be necessary

- the explanation of the variety of therapeutic modalities that may be required and how they fit together within the overall management plan.

  The patient may be required to:

- accept advice on footwear
- undertake exercises such as stretching and strengthening muscles
- consider modification of activity
- lose weight
- have anti-inflammatory therapies such as ultrasound or low-power laser
- actively participate in, and take responsibility for, their own treatment.

PATIENT CONSIDERATIONS

Physical characteristics of the patient must be assessed:

- height, weight and mobility
- the presence of physical disability.

REPLACEABLE PADS

Orthotic therapy often begins with adhesive clinical padding, and the simples extension of such devices to more permanent orthoses are replaceable pads. These devices take many forms:

- plantar pads held in place with elasticised bands positioned around the toes and/or foot. Digital orthoses are held in place with elasticised bands
- silicone orthodigita.

Braces

- Elastic anklets and bracelets – alternative to figure-of-eight strapping when continuing support is required for an unstable rearfoot
- A metatarsal brace is an elastic bandage encircling the metatarsus, often includes a plantar metatarsal pad and may often be combined with a toe loop.

Insoles

Many pathological conditions affecting the plantar surface of the foot can be controlled by appropriate insoles. There are two basic types of insole:

- simple, non-casted, insoles, which essentially act as longer-term padding
- contoured orthoses made to individual or 'averaged' casts/models of the foot.

Manufacture of non-casted insoles

Non-casted insoles are manufactured in such a way that they form part of the shoe. They require:

- the production of a template to the size and shape of the insole of the shoe
- marking of the template with the relevant anatomical landmarks and indication of lesion size and location.

From the wear marks provided on the template appropriate padding can be constructed upon an appropriate base material. The padding is:

- adhered to the base
- covered with leather or synthetic material
- fitted to the shoe.

Casted insoles

Insoles made to a cast may be accommodative or functional orthoses.

Functional orthoses are very popular, and are in routine use in the management of a whole host of disorders of the foot, ankle, lower limbs and even more proximally. There are a number of accepted paradigms which are considered when prescribing a functional orthotic device.

Paradigms in practice: reconciling the controversy of foot function paradigms

The existence of various paradigms fuels deep and prolonged debates amongst enthusiastic academics and clinicians, but may alienate many others. There is clearly a need to resolve these issues in a pragmatic manner that enhances clinical practice and encourages the prescription of orthoses utilising a variety of concepts. Therefore, aiming for a model of practice that uses only one particular model in isolation is unrealistic. It is common, for example, for frontal plane motion control and saggital plane motion facilitation to be incorporated into the same orthoses, so that tissue stresses are reduced. So long as it can be justified based on examination and gait analysis findings, paradigms can be, and routinely are, mixed.

The root paradigm

This focuses on the importance of the subtalar joint (STJ) functioning around the neutral STJ position in promoting optimal function of the foot and lower limb musculoskeletal chain. The focus of the orthoses manufactured from this paradigm characteristically incorporates frontal plane posting to influence the rearfoot and midfoot.

The sagittal plane paradigm

This is based upon the 'rocker theory' proposed by Perry (1992) which asserts that forward progression is dependent upon optimal sagittal plane function around three pivot points ('rockers') in the foot:

- the posterior aspect of the calcaneus
- the ankle joint
- the metatarsophalangeal joints (MTPJs).

It is considered that through sagittal function about these three fulcrums the centre of mass of the body is efficiently transported forward.

The proprioceptive, preferred motion pathway, paradigm

In this model impact forces are considered input signals that 'tune' muscles to modify their activity in the subsequent step to minimise soft-tissue vibration and reduce joint/tendon loading. This paradigm directly challenges motion-control approaches, stating that, although they aim to realign the skeleton, they produce only small changes and the important factor is the influence these orthoses, or shoes, have on muscle activity in terms of their ability to reduce energy cost. This energy cost reduction is the common characteristic of a successful orthosis. The model can be summarised as follows:

- forces acting on the foot during stance act as input signals.
- muscles respond to these signals by modifying their function in the subsequent step.
- the cost function of these adaptations may increase or reduce stress on specific tissues.
- for an intervention to be successful it should support the preferred motion pathway, that is, it should reduce the energy cost and decrease the stress on tissues.
- therefore, orthoses or shoes affect general muscle activity and, therefore, fatigue, comfort, work and performance.

Adapted from Nigg (2001).

The tissue stress paradigm

This paradigm considers that the focus of treatment should not be dominated by a mechanical model, but rather should focus on the presenting pathology, based on the assumption that excess stress was being placed on this tissue. Therefore, the optimal treatment strategy involves reducing this stress by a variety of means. Although the process set out contains several steps, it can be summarised briefly:

- identify the tissue that is painful. This is the tissue that is having excess stress applied to it.
- if it is a mechanical-based problem then shoes/footwear modifications/ orthoses may be useful. However, these should not be made expressly to control motion, but rather to reduce the stresses being applied to the painful tissues.
- in addition to orthoses, other treatments are likely to be indicated. This includes optimising muscle strength, balance and flexibility and using physical therapies to enhance the healing process. Activity modification and a subsequent staged return to activity are also likely to be required.

The tissue stress approach asserts that orthoses are part of a wider treatment approach. An important point is that any orthoses used should provide only the control that is required to reduce stress on the affected tissue to a tolerable level where healing can take place – as opposed to the pursuit of a theoretically ideal position.

Material choice and casting techniques

The choice of materials is dependent on various factors, which include:

- age
- weight
- occupation
- chronicity of the condition where appropriate.

Materials range from rigid to flexible: rigid orthoses provide a higher level of control but, a less rigid material with higher posting might be more comfortable and better tolerated for specific patients. Children normally tolerate semi-rigid or flexible orthoses better than those of the rigid variety.

Range of materials

The most commonly used are:

- carbon fibre composites
- graphite
- polypropylenes and polyethylenes.

Other materials include:

- hexcelite
- aquaplast
- fibreglass fracture-splinting materials.

Temporary functional orthoses

It is possible to manufacture temporary orthoses on the foot using the latter three splinting materials as the temperature required to thermoform devices which are made from them is low.

Custom functional orthoses are manufactured to a model of the patient's foot. The mould or cast is taken using one of a variety of techniques:

- the traditional technique involves laying the patient prone with their foot hanging off the end of the couch and draping plaster of Paris splints over the foot.
- the supine technique can also be used, but control of the foot, which is plantarflexing due to gravity, is more difficult.

Method

- Plaster slabs are draped over the calcaneus and extended down to the forefoot, and brought over the front of the foot and brought up and smoothed into the rearfoot splint.
- They are smoothed together and then the foot is placed in the neutral STJ position where it is held until dry when it can be removed.

The requirement for the STJ to function in neutral is questionable and it may be that all that is required is a cast of the foot moderately less pronated than the functional position.

An alternative technique is to use an oasis foam impression box:

- the patient sits in a chair and the clinician places the foot in a neutral or less pronated position whilst sitting lightly on top of the oasis material, or
- controlled pressure is applied to deform the foam so that it captures the contours of the patient's foot.

In both methods the resulting impression is filled with plaster of Paris which, when set, provides a model of the foot over which the orthosis can be formed.

Additions

Various plaster additions may be incorporated in the plaster model. These include:

- lateral expansions to permit soft tissue spread from the non-weight-bearing casting position
- a forefoot platform which provides functional correction
- medial additions which blend the corrective forefoot platform into the cast.

Moulding

Once heated and malleable, the plastic is trimmed to its rough shape and moulded by vacuum forming until the plastic cools and conforms to the shape and contours of the foot. Different plastics require heating at different temperatures and for different times.

Posting

The type of posting required (intrinsic or extrinsic) should be decided prior to moulding the device. Posts are described as platforms added to the plastic shell to provide correction. An intrinsic post is one that is applied to the cast in the form of a plaster addition or removal so that when the shell is pressed the posting is incorporated into the shell. An extrinsic post involves the addition of material to the bottom of the shell.

Posting materials These are rigid or high-density materials, such as:

- dental acrylic
- tensol (liquid plastic)
- high-density polyethylene
- birkocork.

Posts or wedges hold the foot in the corrected position under load, restrain it from deforming as it would otherwise do, and help restore the normal time sequence of events occurring in the foot during the gait cycle

Rearfoot posts These consist of a shaped wedge placed under the heel of the shell and tapered off on the lateral side to the required angle to control abnormal STJ pronation.

Forefoot posts These may be either varus or valgus, as required, for either inversion or eversion control respectively.

Rigid orthoses thus incorporate all the required correction. However, complete functional control may not always be tolerated at first, and the orthosis should be worn for short periods, increasing daily until they can be worn all day.

Custom versus prefabricated orthoses

Prefabricated devices are available in a range of generic sizes which may satisfy the requirements of patients who:

- have a relatively normal foot size with no or only minor deformity
- require a moderate amount of intrinsic control.

Evidence is emerging concerning prefabricated orthoses to suggest they may offer, in a number of circumstances, equivalent therapeutic value to bespoke devices. Prefabricated orthoses would seem to offer potential and certainly should not be ignored.

Computer-aided design and manufacture orthoses

The computer-aided design and manufacture (CAD–CAM) of functional orthoses is now recognised by many in the profession as the way forward, enabling practitioners to prescribe and supply their patients with devices that are produced to much finer tolerances than those available through the traditional hand-crafted methods.

The data for the design is obtained from a neutral plaster cast of the patient's foot or the foot itself may be scanned. Good-quality casts of the type best suited to the laboratory's specification are essential, as is the quality and clarity of the prescription, to enable the manufacturer to produce the correct devices.

The prescription data are retained on the laboratories' data bank, enabling repeat prescriptions to be produced at any time. Most laboratories are willing to provide expert help to practitioners with their casting technique and prescription writing.

Factors that influence the choice of functional device prescribed

- Footwear – This is often a problem for female patients who need to wear a dress or court shoe for social or occupational reasons.
- Occupation – The requirement to wear safety footwear must also be considered.

Types of functional orthoses

- Standard – Normal shell incorporating all postings and accommodation
- Gait plate – The distal edge of the device is extended beyond the 4th and 5th metatarsal heads, to function as a counterirritant. Some practitioners use it to treat gait problems

- Heel skives (Kirby skive) – The Kirby skive is a cast modification that involves angulating the medial 1/3 of the heel cup to produce a heel cup that is inclined to provide an effective anti-pronatory force.

Problems associated with fitting functional orthoses

- Devices do not fit shoes
- Devices cut into the lateral side of the heel
- 1st metatarsal irritation
- Devices are too tight at the heel
- Irritation in the area of the medial longitudinal arch
- Insufficient control.

All of these problems can be dealt with by the experienced practitioner and further guidance is available in *Neale's Disorders of the Foot*.

Heel orthoses

There are a number of orthoses which may be made specifically for conditions affecting the heel. A heel cup may be fabricated on a cast of the heel using plastics already described, or fibreglass. Such devices are well tolerated because they take up little room and can be worn in a wide variety of shoes. Wedges or posts may be incorporated into such devices at the time of manufacture or at a later stage.

These devices are corrective in nature. However, palliative heel orthoses may be required for lesions on the plantar aspect of the heel. Such heel orthoses can be manufactured on casts or made directly onto the heel using silicone.

Latex technique

Deformities of the toes, such as hallux abductovalgus and hammer toes, are often chronic and require protection more or less permanently. In such cases, devices made in latex are often the most effective type of orthosis. Such techniques are now rarely used, but represent a rewarding technique for patient and podiatrist alike.

Digital appliances for the lesser toes

Latex techniques may be used for lesser toe devices; however, nowadays direct-moulding techniques utilising silicone rubbers or thermoplastic materials are more commonly used. Silicone rubbers are well proven as the most suitable materials for digital orthoses. They can also be fabricated from orthotic plastic, but it is then usually necessary to line them with softer material for good tissue tolerance.

Silicones

Silicones are generally presented as a putty-like substance, to which a catalyst is added. After a period, the putty is transformed into a flexible solid. The material, while undergoing its change of state, maintains a putty-like consistency for a period ranging from 2 to 8 minutes, depending on the putty:catalyst ratio and the room temperature. This space of time allows the practitioner to fabricate the device.

Correction of deformity

Silicone orthodigita may be used to:

- correct congenital digital deformities in children
- correct toe deformities in older patients, if sufficient motion is present in the affected joints
- maintain correction following corrective digital surgery.

Basically, the splint is fashioned around the toes, and, as the silicone sets, the toes are held in their corrected position until the elastic properties of the material are strong enough to withstand the deforming forces.

Thermoplastics

These are usually products of additional polymerisation. They will soften on heating and harden once cooled without any chemical change taking place. Polymers which are thermoplastic can be moulded to a desired shape when heat and pressure are applied.

This range of synthetic materials has four main areas of application:

- firm splinting
- impression medium
- moulded lining
- modelling and construction.

The firm splinting material is polyethylene sheet, which may be used for direct moulding to positive casts in the production of orthotic shells.

The impression material is the expanded polyethylene which, when inserted into the shoe as a template insole, provides an accurate dynamic impression of pressure areas.

The two most commonly used thermoplastics are expanded vinyl acetate (EVA) and expanded polyethylene (Plastozote). After it is heated, the thermoplastic is moulded directly onto the foot and additional padding and outer layers are added in sequence.

Footwear which conforms accurately to the shape of the foot can be simply constructed using these materials using the various densities and thicknesses. Such devices include:

- clogs with an enclosed front and no heel counter
- sandals with a block sole and two or three straps to hold it on to the foot.

These and more complicated styles can also be produced, which, when compared with traditional surgical footwear, are extremely attractive in terms of weight, fitting, style and price.

'Hot water plastics' (polyform, aquaplast hexcelite (x-lite plus)

These are of particular use when an immediate appliance is required, and this technique is of great value in saving the practitioner time. Its essential features are:

- low-temperature moulding
- chairside technique
- production time of a few minutes
- rapid remoulding of part of or the whole device
- minimal waste material.

CONCLUSION

As can be seen from the number of techniques described, it is inappropriate to think of the term 'orthosis' as describing a narrow range of devices dominated by simple and functional insoles and silicone wedges. Podiatrists have a rich history of skilful manufacture of a range of devices and it is vital, for the management of idiosyncratic and challenging patients and rewarding practice, that practitioners embrace a range of techniques.

Chapter | 16 |

Footwear

Assessment and evaluation of footwear is an essential component of the podiatric management of foot and lower-limb problems. The relationship between the foot, lower-limb pathologies, foot function and the resultant gait within footwear may be complex, but an understanding of all these components is required for the maximum effective podiatric management. *Therapeutic footwear* is a valuable aid to any therapy designed to improve foot health. Footwear alone can resolve the consequences of many biomechanical anomalies, aid joint function and reduce friction and pressure to which the foot might otherwise be subjected. Effective footwear advice and prescription (if required) is essential.

FUNCTIONS OF FOOTWEAR

- Primary function:
  - protection
- Secondary functions:
  - complementing an outfit
  - fashion
  - occupation – corporate image, armed forces
  - conducting specific tasks – dancing
  - compensating for an abnormality.

FOOTWEAR STYLES

There are various footwear styles which are worn dependent on the activity for which the shoe will be used. Each style can be adapted with variations to reflect fashion trends.

- Lacing shoe. This style holds the foot firmly within the shoe and is the preferred style recommended by podiatrists

- Oxford shoe. A decorative version of this shoe is the brogue. This shoe has normally five pairs of eyelets and fits closely over the dorsal plantar area of the foot. This close apposition means that this style may not be suitable for a high-arched foot.
- Derby shoe. Also referred to as a Gibson shoe. This shoe is suitable for a high-arched or a broad foot.
- Moccasin-style shoe. Can be slip on or lacing. Suitable for people with good foot function. Stitching of the 'apron front' of this style of shoe results in internal seams and can cause pressure on deformities such as hallux abductovalgus or lesser toe deformities.
- Sandal. Strapless (mules) and sling-back sandals rely on relatively ineffective straps on the dorsal aspect of the foot or round the heel to hold the foot in the footwear. If worn habitually various stresses are applied to the foot and give rise to callous formation on the plantar aspect of the foot and round the rim of the heel. There is poor stability of the foot within the footwear. Enclosed sandals may have many of the desirable features of a shoe incorporated.
- Court shoe. Prolonged wear of this type of shoe results in poor fit with the foot poorly retained and resultant friction and pressure occurs.
- Sports shoes. A wide variety is commercially available with the particular features incorporated specific to the sporting activity. This type of footwear can be recommended for regular wear as they have many desirable features of a good-fitting shoe.
- Boots. These are used by a variety of professions including the police, armed forces, fire fighters, land workers, etc., and may include Wellington boots.
- Fashion boots are worn by both sexes, but styles vary from those which have good fitting and retention for the foot to those which are a fashion statement and are totally unsuitable for a foot with pathologies.

CLASSES OF THERAPEUTIC FOOTWEAR

Therapeutic footwear may be classed under several categories.

- Normal retail footwear – modified as required
- Stock surgical footwear – manufacturers provide low-cost stock ranges. Colours are black or brown. Wide range of sizes and fittings. The measurements given include size, length, width at the metatarsophalangeal joints (MTPJ), girth at the MTPJ and instep girth
- Modular footwear – prescribed for feet which cannot be accommodated from stock ranges. Made from manufacturer's existing last with limited modifications. Additional width, girth height and length can be added.
- Bespoke footwear requires a new last. Made by plaster of Paris impressions of feet and lower legs and charting a diagram of the foot outline with length, width and girth measurements identified at specific points on each foot.

Conditions which may benefit from therapeutic footwear prescription include:

- cases where foot shape and function vary from the normal due to congenital abnormality, trauma or surgical intervention
- patients with scarring as a result of leg ulcers, burns, tissue grafts and muscle flap repairs to debriding injuries may develop contractures and may have an altered gait pattern
- long-term bulky dressings or lower limb or foot oedema

- limb-length discrepancy
- peripheral vascular disease with atrophy of skin and nail in the foot
- diabetes when the complications of the disease have affected the feet
- abnormal gait and impaired mobility
- severe painful hallux valgus, hallux rigidus, pes cavus, toe deformities
- all types of connective tissue disorders, arthritic conditions.

PARTS OF THE SHOE

Component parts of the upper

- Toe box. The most anterior part of a shoe. Accommodates the toes. The toe puff maintains the shape of the toe box. Protection of the toes is achieved by steel toe protectors in industrial footwear. Poor length or breadth in this component will cause compression of the toes.
- Toe cap. This is at the toe end of the shoe. In normal footwear protection by the toe cap is negligible and is mainly used to provide strength and wear to the area.
- Vamp. Anteriorly this is attached to the toe cap and posteriorly to the quarters. This part of the shoe is subjected to flexion during gait (MTPJ forms the fulcrum point of the foot) particularly at the propulsive phase. A flexible material is required such as leather as it is capable of withstanding repeated stress.
- Tongue. The main function of this component is protection from laces, eyelets and straps. The tongue also absorbs pressure to protect the dorsum of the foot when the laces are firmly tied and straps are firmly pulled in place.
- Quarters. The posterior part of the shoe and consists of medial and lateral components. A close fit to the tarsal and metatarsal area holds the foot firmly within the shoe when correctly laced. The addition of a counter to the quarters adds strength to the shoe and minimises mediolateral movement of the heel of the foot within the shoe and maximises normal foot and joint function during stance and gait preventing a variety of bone and soft-tissue pathologies. Fig 16.1

Component parts of the sole

- Insole. Should be smooth, may contain padding material (particularly sports shoes) which can be removed to insert orthoses if required
- Bottom fillings are traditionally made of cork in the Oxford shoes. This allows a slight compression, which permits an accommodative depression particularly below the metatarsal heads. Modern shoes may not contain bottom fillings
- Welt. Joining material uniting the upper to the outsole. Usually in the Oxford and other more expensive shoes
- Outsole. Is in direct contact with the ground. May be leather, rubber, crepe or synthetic hard-wearing material. Should be flexible for gait particularly propulsion. Some materials provide more shock absorption than others. Leather is a poor shock absorber; rubber, crepe and some synthetic materials provide better shock absorption, protecting the foot against impact and ground reaction force.

Uppers

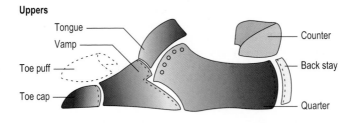

Sole

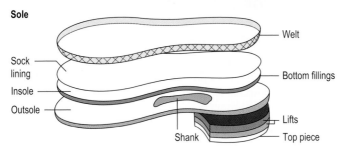

Figure 16.1 Parts of the shoe based on the traditional Oxford shoe.

Subsidiary parts

- Heel
- Shank
- Counter
- Backstay.

FEATURES OF A GOOD-FITTING SHOE/THERAPEUTIC FOOTWEAR

- A good retaining medium: laces or Velcro straps capable of holding the shoe onto the foot.
- Close-fitting medial and lateral quarters are important to hold the foot firmly in the shoe; the quarters should be one piece of material with no back seam to irritate the retrocalcaneal area. Leather is the most popular material and the one which suits most foot pathologies but occasionally there is a need to use an extensible material such as neoprene.
- Toe puff – a toe rim which holds the shoe up over the toe area is required. A standard toe puff covers the area at the front of the vamp as far proximally as the interphalangeal joints (IPJs) or can be reinforced to give additional protection against trauma. In the presence of sensory neuropathy and deformed toes the rim toe puff is indicated to hold up the front of the shoe, but not extend proximally over the dorsum of the toes. The toes will be protected by the upper and lining material without the added hardness of toe puff material in this area.
- Without any stiffening shoes will collapse, crease and cause damage to the feet. Without heel counters the shoe quarters will collapse and the shoe may slip off the foot.
- The vamp should be seam-free and any pattern or decoration should be added externally as internal seams may irritate.

- There should be adequate width and depth in the toe box to accommodate any toe deformities.
- The shoe must be the correct length to prevent impingement of the toes and various nail conditions caused by trauma.
- The shoe must be the correct width fitting. The widest part of the shoe should correspond to the widest part of the foot which is normally transversely between the 1st and 5th metatarsal heads.
- There should be an adequate heel seat. This should accommodate the width of the heel without being too wide, which leads to movement of the heel within the shoes and may cause diffuse heel callous. In severe cases this results in plantar calcaneal bursitis and the development of footstrain. If the heel seat is too narrow this may cause 'wedging' of the heel and a ridge of callous on the peripheral plantar aspect of the heel.
- The extent of the heel counter and the support provided should be evaluated. Patients with ankle instability may find a boot helpful with heel counters additionally stiffened and extended proximally through the quarter. In a mid foot deformity, particularly a valgus deformity, the quarters may be extended distally through to the waist of the shoe. This will minimise deformation of the shoe during gait and can also be used to reinforce the action of an orthosis.
- Heel height should be no greater than 5 cm (2 inches). Increased heel height increases the load on the forefoot causing foot pathologies and extends the lumbar spine to maintain upright posture and good balance leading to lower back problems. Certain pathologies require the prescription of a higher than normal heel height, e.g. the effect of surgical intervention on ankle mobility. Ankle joint fixation may vary from the normal 90° and the required heel height will be affected.
- There should be a broad heel base in contact with the ground which gives stability. A narrow heel base leads to instability and increases the risk of inversion ankle sprains or fractures.
- The upper material should be made of leather as it is flexible to permit movement and permeable to perspiration.
- With respect to the sole and heel leather has some disadvantages: it has poor slip resistance in wet conditions, has little effect in reducing the magnitude of ground reaction force against the foot, and absorbs and retains water when wet underfoot conditions are present.
- A range of materials for outsole units specifically indicated for certain types of activity are available, including polymers, most commonly polyurethane, thermoplastic rubber and EVA (ethylene vinyl acetate). These have good shock absorption. The viscosity and elasticity of the outsole are important factors in reducing the magnitude of ground reaction force against the foot. The co-efficient of friction of the outsole material is important. It should allow the foot to move easily across the surface without slipping and without gripping the ground surface too firmly to prevent falls.
- Studies on safety footwear showed that the characteristics of the floor/sole combination, occupation and activities must be considered when prescribing. A rough terrain requires commando soles with additional grip. A lightweight, smooth-surfaced outsole and heel is ideal for a lightweight person with a shuffling gait.

FOOTWEAR AND LAST TERMINOLOGY

- Tread line. This runs from the 1st to the 5th metatarsal heads and corresponds to the widest part of the forefoot.

- Toe spring. The toe spring reduces the amount of flexion required at the MTPJs during propulsion and reduces foot fatigue. A high toe spring can be seen in a wooden clog.
- Rigidity of outsole. A shoe with a rigid sole incorporates a high toe spring to permit propulsion. A thin-soled shoe has less toe spring.
- Heel height. This also influences the height of the toe spring.
- Heel pitch. This is the angle of elevation of the heel seat of the last from the horizontal surface. Heel pitch is dependent on the heel height.
- Flare. The flare of a shoe can be established by drawing a line from the centre of the heel seat forward through the sole of the shoe. Measuring from the treadline if there is a greater area of sole on the medial side then this would be an in-flare shoe. Conversely a greater area of sole on the lateral side of the tread is an out-flare shoe. An equal amount of sole is a straight-flare shoe. A pes plano valgus foot represents an 'out-flare' foot and a pes cavus a 'straight flare' foot. The foot and shoe should have corresponding flares.

DESIRABLE FOOTWEAR FEATURES FOR SPECIFIC FOOT CONDITIONS

The podiatrist should recommend footwear in relation to the presenting foot condition.

Hallux abductovalgus

- Additional 'bunion' pocket to accommodate the joint
- Seam-free uppers with no stitching to irritate the 1st and 5th metatarsal heads
- Deep toe box to accommodate lesser toe deformities.

Hallux limitus/rigidus

- Seam-free uppers with no stitching to irritate the enlarged 1st MTPJ on the dorsal aspect
- Thick outsole with high toe spring to compensate for reduced range of movement at 1st MTPJ
- Removable insoles to allow fitting of bespoke orthoses
- Deep toe box to accommodate enlarged 1st MTPJ.

Short broad foot

- Derby-style shoe with wide opening anterior quarters
- Broad, padded tongue under eyelets
- Thick shock-absorbing outsole
- Exaggerated high toe-spring
- Good heel-to-ball fitting
- Good depth to shoe
- Rounded toe box to accommodate digital formulae
- Removable insole to allow fitting of bespoke orthoses.

Long mobile foot

- Narrow fitting
- Close-fitting rear quarters and counters

- Good retaining medium
- Good heel-to-ball fitting.

High-arched foot

- May need slightly higher heel than standard footwear
- Derby-style shoe with wide opening anterior quarters
- Fully adjustable laces joining the quarters
- Broad, padded tongue
- Deep toe box which is well rounded to accommodate digital formulae
- Thick shock-absorbing outsole
- Exaggerated high toe spring
- Good posterior and forepart depth to shoe
- Good heel-to-ball fitting
- Removable insole to allow fitting of bespoke orthoses.

Rheumatoid foot

- Broad heel base with medial buttress
- Upper and outsole of a lightweight robust construction
- Wedged outsole
- Lightweight, thick pressure-absorbing outsole
- Straight flare is often required (out-flare in advanced disease)
- Seamless forepart to uppers – no stitching
- Self-adhering 'hook and loop' broad retaining strap
- Well-cushioned tongue
- Close-fitting quarters
- Removable insole to allow fitting of bespoke orthoses
- Soft, smooth, hardwearing inner lining to uppers.

Diabetic foot

- Removable, thick, pressure-absorbing insoles to permit fitting of bespoke orthoses
- Seam-free uppers with no stitching
- Upper and outsole of a light, robust construction
- Good retaining medium
- Well-padded tongue, which is a continuation of the vamp
- Soft, smooth, hardwearing inner lining to uppers
- Thick pressure-absorbing outsole.

WEAR MARKS AS AN AID TO DIAGNOSIS

Examination of the wear marks on the upper and sole of shoes is a good aid to confirming diagnosis of foot function and no clinical examination should be considered complete until the footwear has been fully examined. Wear marks should not be considered as standard; however, certain abnormalities and gait patterns do tend to present with typical patterns of wear. As a guide, typical wear patterns seen in the 'normal' foot and contrasted with those seen in association with common foot abnormalities are summarised below.

Normal wear

- The outsole and heel.
  - Posterior/lateral heel wear
  - Heavier wear across forepart of sole at tread line becoming more apparent in the area of the 1st and 2nd metatarsal head
  - Heavier wear distal to the 1st metatarsal head corresponding to toe-off by the hallux.
- The insole (sock lining).
  - Uniform discoloration of the heel seat only slightly greater on the posterior/lateral border
  - Lateral discoloration of the waist of the insole corresponding to the soft tissue of the lateral longitudinal arch
  - Discoloration and some indentation at the metatarsal heads. This may be slightly more evident under the central and 1st metatarsal heads
  - Distal discoloration corresponding to the pulps of the toes approximately 1 cm from the distal end of the shoe.
- The lining of the upper.
  - The lining at the posterior aspect of the quarters, corresponding to the backstay, and that of the medial and lateral quarters should be evenly discoloured.
  - The lining of the distal end of the toe box and the toe puff should be smooth with no evidence of indentation or undue wear.
- The upper.
  - In welted shoes, when viewed directly from above, no part of the upper of the forepart should obscure the welt.
  - The main transverse crease across the vamp should be mildly oblique corresponding to the metatarsal formula and be consistent with the appearance of the tread line of the outsole.
  - Anterior quarters should be parallel and directly oppose one another.
  - Medial and lateral quarters should be symmetrical.
  - Material of upper should be essentially smooth and evenly contoured with no obvious distortion.

Wear marks seen in association with common foot disorders

Hallux limitus/rigidus

- The outsole and heel.
  - Excessive posterior/lateral heel wear
  - Heavy wear under the 5th metatarsal head. This may display evidence of internal rotation of the limb through the appearance of wear marks appearing as concentric rings
  - Wear under the 2nd metatarsal head may be exaggerated
  - Minimal wear under the 1st metatarsal head
  - The height of the toe spring may be reduced
  - Excessive wear may be evident on the under surface corresponding to the distal phalanx of the hallux
- The insole (sock lining).
  - Excessive discoloration on lateral border of heel seat
  - Heavy discoloration and depression of bottom fillings in the region of the 5th metatarsal head; may also present as excessive wear of insole material
  - Heavy discoloration and depression of bottom fillings under the central metatarsal heads and, particularly, the second

- Minimal discoloration and depression under the 1st metatarsal head
- Deep depression and discoloration under the distal phalanx of the hallux; may also present as excessive wearing of insole material
- Deep depression and discoloration of insole from toe pulp of lesser toes
- The lining of the upper.
  - Lateral lining of the quarters exhibits excessive wear
  - Excessive wear of lateral lining of the vamp in the region of the 5th MTPJ
  - Excessive wear of lining of the medial/dorsal vamp consistent with excessive wear in the area from osteophyte formation at the 1st MTPJ
- The upper.
  - Evidence of bulging of the posterior/lateral quarters over the outsole at the heel
  - Lateral vamp may bulge over the outsole consistent with prolonged inversion of hindfoot and forefoot
  - Shallow dorsal creasing of the vamp is diagonal from the 5th MTPJ to a point just lateral to the 1st MTPJ
  - Diagonal dorsal creasing of the vamp gives way to dorsal bulging of the upper to accommodate dorsal exostosis formation at the 1st MTPJ
  - The throat of the shoe may appear to drift laterally.

Pes cavus

- The outsole and heel.
  - Heavy transverse wear at posterior aspect of heel
  - Heavy wear across tread line
  - Minimal wear proximal and distal to tread line
  - Toe spring of shoe may be exaggerated
- The insole (sock lining).
  - Heavy discoloration and wear on heel seat
  - Extreme discoloration, depression of bottom fillings and excessive wear across area in contact with metatarsal heads
  - If claw toes are present there may be a deep discoloration and depression corresponding to the toe pulps
- The lining of the upper.
  - The lining of the medial, lateral and posterior quarters may show evidence of excessive wear
  - The lining of the tongue may be depressed and show evidence of excessive wear due to the prominent tarsal bones
  - The lining of the upper toe box may show excessive wear due to the pressure applied by the clawed or retracted toes and the retraction of the hallux
- The upper.
  - The posterior quarters may bulge over the outsole due to the fullness of the heel
  - The anterior quarters show stretching due to the prominence of the tarsal region; when shoes are on the feet there may be a failure of the anterior quarters to parallel and correctly oppose one another
  - There may be a deep transverse crease across the vamp
  - Bulging of the upper anterior to the vamp accommodating severely clawed or retracted toes
  - Tongue may not display evidence of eyelet compression; only lace marks may be evident due to failure of anterior quarters to adequately oppose one another. Consequently, the dorsal aspect of the foot is not adequately protected from the eyelets.

Pes planovalgus

- The outsole and heel.
  - Posterior/lateral heel wear
  - Anterior/medial heel wear
  - Waist of shoe may collapse and be in ground contact
  - Shank may break and penetrate the waist of shoe
  - Excessive wear under 2nd, 3rd and 4th metatarsal heads
  - Excessive wear anterior/medial aspect of forepart of shoe
- The insole (sock lining).
  - Excessive wear of insole and sock lining under 2nd, 3rd and 4th metatarsal heads
  - Wear on insole may be more apparent on medial aspect at the waist of shoe when compared to the lateral aspect
  - Excessive wear at the forepart of the insole relative to the pulps of the lesser toes; in particular the 3rd, 4th and 5th as they are forced into a clawed position through impact against the toe box due to the associated abduction of the forefoot
- The lining of the upper.
  - Excessive wear of lining of lateral toe box
  - Excessive wear of anterior/medial aspect of toe box lining due to impaction of hallux
  - Posterior medial and lateral quarters may demonstrate excessive wear
- The upper.
  - Medial drifting of the throat of shoe
  - Posterior and lateral quarters appear excessively wide and rounded
  - Medial quarters bulge over outsole
  - Shallow transverse crease marks on vamp
  - If secondary hallux abductovalgus is present, bulging of the quarters on the medial side of the vamp will be noted. Bulging of lateral toe box secondary to clawing of the lesser toes of the abducted forefoot.

FOOTWEAR MODIFICATIONS

Prior to prescribing therapeutic (orthopaedic) footwear, foot size, foot shape and biomechanical function are assessed. Footwear purchased from a retail outlet should be considered for modification. If the footwear is of suitable style and material a number of adaptations can be made. For example, a ball and ring stretcher can be used to stretch leather uppers to accommodate problems such as toe deformities and hallux abductovalgus; tongue pads and heel grips can be included to improve fit. Despite these options there will be a small number of patients whose foot health needs can only be accommodated in specialist footwear.

Heel modifications

- The SACH heel (solid ankle cushion heel). The posterior portion is replaced by a softer material which reduces shock at heel strike and compensates for reduced ankle joint motion.
- Thomas heel. This has an anterior medial extension of the heel by 0.5 inch designed to give additional support to the sustentaculum tali and medial longitudinal arch. A lateral or reverse Thomas heel supports the cuboid and tends to rotate the foot externally.

- Flared heels (floats) add leverage to control the heel. A grossly inverted heel indicates a lateral flare to stabilise the ankle and subtalar joint (STJ), a medial heel flare is indicated if the strike is too everted.
- Combined heel and sole modifications.

Wedges

- Medial heel and sole wedges are prescribed when the medial aspect of the foot bears too much weight.
- Lateral heel wedges with anterior extensions transfer weight off the 5th metatarsal shaft.
- Contralateral wedging includes a medial heel extension or wedge (e.g. Thomas heel) and a lateral forefoot wedge.
- Through-sole and heel wedging gives greater stability during gait.
- Lateral sole wedges transfer weight from the lateral to the medial side of the shoe.
- Medial toe wedges discourage in-toeing but should be used with caution.

Bars

Metatarsal bars may be added posterior to the metatarsal heads on the outer sole of shoes to help in off-loading metatarsal heads.

Rocker soles

Characterised by a rigid sole which restricts movement at the joints metatarsophalangeal joints. Walking in the rigid shoe is possible because the shoe tips forward when the centre of pressure moves distal to the rocker fulcrum. In some cases this can lead to a negative heel where the heel is functioning at a lower level than the treadline foot position. Rocker soles eliminate the propulsive phase of gait. Unloading in the rocker soled shoe may be a combination of the following effects:

- redistribution of load over a larger area
- increase in the loading time for the regions of the foot in contact with the rigid shoe
- change in the function of the foot due to restriction of motion particularly at the MTPJs
- change in the patterns of motion of the lower extremity due to the altered geometry and rigidity of the shoe
- reduction in shear pressure on the plantar surface.

Shoe raises

Shoe raises added to the outer sole compensate for limb-length discrepancy. Individuals with limb-length discrepancy may use specific strategies to improve ambulation. Full compensation is not always acceptable/comfortable initially and it is better to under-prescribe the raise height and evaluate again at a later prescription. A limb-length discrepancy of 4 cm should have a raise of 4 cm placed under the heel, 2 cm under the MTPJs tapering to either 1 cm or 0 cm at the toe depending on the length of the foot and the degree of angulation required for forward propulsion.

Types of raises

- Heel elevation contained inside footwear may be used where the elevation required is <1 cm. Raises may be made of cork, EVA of high shore value

(70 shore) or of materials of similar density. Surgical footwear may have deeper quarters to include the raise. An internal and external raise may be used on the same shoe, splitting the height of the raise required between the internal and external raises.

- External raises can be added to existing soles if the soling and heel material are suitable. A heel raise only will affect the heel-height and toe spring relationship and the shoe will no longer stand correctly on its tread line.

ASSESSING THE FIT OF THERAPEUTIC FOOTWEAR

Whether fitting new therapeutic footwear or evaluating the effectiveness of existing therapeutic footwear the effectiveness of the fit should always be assessed. Therapeutic footwear is normally provided with a selection of inlays which match the width and length of the shoe and which provide a useful tool to assess the dimensions of the shoe in comparison with the foot:

- check the overall length of the inlay from the back of the heel to the longest toe
- check the heel to ball length
- check that the MTPJs are positioned at the widest part of the inlay
- check the ball-to-toe length.

If the above lengths are not appropriate the shoe will never fit properly. With the shoe on the foot, including any orthoses to be worn note the following:

- the way in which the foot slips into the shoe. This often indicates how well the shoe will fit, but the shoe must be fastened to evaluate fit.
- examine for a good snug heel fit because the way the foot is held back in the shoe determines the position of the foot within the shoe.
- ensure the counter is not causing pressure on the maleoli or the back of the heel.
- check the fastenings of the shoe and ensure that the facings are lined up correctly.
- look at the instep area and ensure that fit is neither too tight nor too loose.
- evaluate girth and depth at the MTPJs and over the toes.
- ensure that there are no bony prominences visible or evident on palpation which could be damaged by a too-shallow vamp or toe area in the shoe.
- the patient should walk in the shoe to ensure there is no heel slippage and stability in gait is evident.

CONCLUSION

Footwear is not only a fashion item or a protection for the feet. In its various forms footwear can facilitate activity, improve mobility, become an effective therapy, reduce morbidity, and improve and extend a quality life. To ensure that footwear is optimal the podiatrist needs to understand how the normal foot functions when shod, how the shoe may have contributed to any pathology present and conversely how the various components of the shoe may be used to remedy any pathological state. Footwear should be regarded as part of both diagnostic and therapeutic strategies.

Chapter 17

Pain control

Pain is a common cause of limp and needs to be diagnosed and managed appropriately. Pain control is required in the acute setting, after surgery or trauma for instance. Pain is a fundamental component of the stress response to injury and if it is not adequately controlled it can impede the recovery process and result in complications (Table 17.1). Pain also persists in many chronic conditions which affect the foot (Table 17.2).

DEFINITION

The International Association for the Study of Pain (IASP) defines pain as 'an unpleasant sensory and emotional experience associated with potential or actual tissue damage'. Pain is a complex interaction of sensory, emotional and behavioural factors, and, therefore, its diagnosis and treatment must address all of these aspects. Pain is classified into nociceptive, neuropathic and psychogenic; all can be either acute or chronic. Acute somatic pain is the most common type of pain that podiatrists will deal with in clinical practice.

ANATOMY

- Pain is transmitted from the peripheral tissues to the brain cortex via three distinct levels; called primary, secondary and tertiary afferents.
- Peripheral pain receptors or nociceptors are activated to produce an action potential.
- The action potential conducts along the primary afferent nerve fibres (peripheral level) to synapse with secondary afferent fibres (spinal level) which ascend up the spinal cord.
- The impulse then synapses to tertiary afferents within various structures in the brain (supra-spinal level).
- Optimal analgesia can only be obtained by utilising treatments which work via different mechanisms and pathways.

Table 17.1 Pathophysiological associations of pain

ORGAN SYSTEM	POTENTIAL EFFECTS
Central nervous system	Inhumane, misery, anxiety, depression, sleep disturbance
Cardiovascular system	↑ blood pressure, heart rate and vascular resistance, ↑ cardiac ischaemia
Respiratory system	Cough inhibition (pneumonia), hyperventilation (respiratory alkalosis)
Gastrointestinal system	Ileus, nausea, vomiting
Genitourinary system	Urinary retention, uterine inhibition
Muscle	Restless – ↑ oxygen consumption Immobility – ↑ incidence of pulmonary thromboembolism
Metabolic	↑ Catabolic: cortisone, glucagon, growth hormone, catecholamines ↓ Anabolic: insulin, testosterone ↑ Plasminogen activator inhibitor (↑ blood clotting)

SOMATIC PAIN

- *Physiological* pain, also known as first or 'fast' pain, is a protective and useful event which enables the organism to rapidly and accurately localise pain and withdraw from the stimulus in order to avoid or reduce further tissue damage. It is produced by stimulation of *high threshold thermo/mechanical nociceptors* and is transmitted by fast-conducting A delta (Aδ) fibres. The Aδ primary afferent enters the dorsal horn of the spinal cord and synapses at laminae I, V and X. Conduction continues along the secondary afferent fibres via the neospinothalamic tract which is monosynaptic as it ascends to the *posterior thalamic nuclei* (Fig 17.1). From there it synapses with tertiary afferents to the somatosensory post-central gyrus at the cortex. If this short-duration stimulus does not result in tissue damage, the pain disappears when the stimulus stops.
- *Pathophysiological* pain, sometimes called second or 'slow' pain is responsible for the delayed pain sensation that occurs after tissue injury and which encourages tissue healing by eliciting behaviour designed to protect the damaged area. This is the type of pain that occurs after surgery, trauma and inflammation, and is the kind which health carers strive to manage in the clinical setting.
- In addition to the two types of nociceptors mentioned above, there are 'silent' or 'sleeping' nociceptors. They are present in the skin and visceral organs and become active under inflammatory conditions.

PHYSIOLOGY

Peripheral nociceptor level

- Most pain originates from tissue damage. The release of inflammatory mediators from tissues, immune cells and sympathetic and sensory afferent

Table 17.2 Characteristics of clinical pain

NOCICEPTIVE: (PAIN DUE TO TISSUE DAMAGE)

	Somatic (skin, bone, muscle – OA, RA, ulceration, infection)	Visceral (sympathetically innervated organs)
Site	Well-localised, cutaneous or deep	Vague distribution
Radiation	Dermatomal	Diffuse, can be transferred to body surface
Character	Sharp, aching, throbbing, gnawing	Dull, vague (cramping, squeezing, dragging)
Periodicity	Often constant, also incident pain	Often periodic, building up to peaks
Associations	Rarely	Nausea/vomiting, sweaty Blood pressure and heart rate changes

NEUROPATHIC: (PAIN DUE TO INJURY OF NERVE FIBRES OR TRACTS)

Site of injury	Central – post stroke central pain, phantom limb pain Mixed – plexus avulsion, post herpetic neuralgia Peripheral – neuroma, nerve compression, neuralgias, painful diabetic polyneuropathy, complex regional pain syndrome
Character	Burning, tingling, pricking, numb, cold, pressing, squeezing, itching Constant and/or intermittent shooting, lancinating, electric shock

PSYCHOGENIC:

Pain entirely due to psychological or psychiatric pathology is rare. One-third of medically depressed patients will have pain as one of their primary complaints but this will resolve as their depression is managed

Anxiety and depression are common sequelae of severe and chronic pain and often contribute to the unpleasant experience of pain. They need to be managed in conjunction as pain management will be less successful if they are not

OA = osteoarthritis, RA = rheumatoid arthritis

nerve fibres results in an 'inflammatory soup' bathing the nociceptors. This sensitisation to pain is called *allodynia* when it is produced by normally non-painful stimulation, such as touch.

Spinal level

- The dorsal horn area of the spinal cord is the site where complex interconnections occur between excitatory and inhibitory interneurons and the descending inhibitory tracts from the brain.

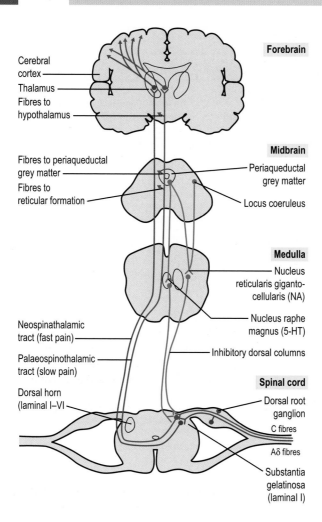

Cerebral cortex
Thalamus
Fibres to hypothalamus

Forebrain

Fibres to periaqueductal grey matter
Fibres to reticular formation

Midbrain

Periaqueductal grey matter
Locus coeruleus

Medulla

Nucleus reticularis giganto-cellularis (NA)
Nucleus raphe magnus (5-HT)

Neospinathalamic tract (fast pain)
Palaeospinothalamic tract (slow pain)

Inhibitory dorsal columns

Spinal cord

Dorsal horn (laminal I–VI

Dorsal root ganglion
C fibres
Aδ fibres
Substantia gelatinosa (laminal I)

Ascending nociceptive fast (red) and slow (green) pathways.
Descending inhibitory tracts (yellow).
NA, noradrenaline; 5-HT, 5 hydroxytryptamine;

Figure 17.1 Spinal and supraspinal pathways of pain.

- Excitatory amino acids and neuropeptides are the neurotransmitters involved in the nociceptive transmission through the dorsal horn.

Supra-spinal level

- The supra-spinal organisation and function in nociception is highly complex but the perception of pain is associated with changes in activity of the thalamus, primary and secondary cortex, and, particularly, the anterior cingulate cortex.
- The descending inhibitory dorsal column pathways originate at the level of the cortex and thalamus.

Neuropathic pain

- Neuropathic pain occurs following damage to the neural structures. When the damage is only partial, gross motor and sensory function can be preserved and nerve activity can often be increased. This can result in subtle abnormalities, such as altered temperature sensation, unusual or unpleasant feelings, or even pain. This may occur after surgery on the toes, resulting in an interdigital neuroma, or with medical conditions such as diabetes or shingles.
- Patients often find neuropathic pain symptoms difficult to describe, but some of the words commonly used include burning, tingling, numb, pressing, squeezing and itching (Table 17.2). The pain can be constant or intermittent, and may be associated with electric shooting sensations. Examples of neuropathic pain affecting the lower limbs include:
  - painful diabetic neuropathy
  - post-operative neuromas
  - entrapment neuropathies
  - some types of complex regional pain syndrome (CRPS).
- It is important to identify any treatable aetiology of pain in order to prevent progression of the disease.

PRINCIPLES OF PAIN MANAGEMENT

- The general principle of pain management is based on managing the component parts of the condition, namely the nociceptive and neuropathic constituents.
- Pain symptoms are managed with techniques which fall into four main groups:
  - pharmacological
  - regional analgesia
  - physical therapy
  - psychological therapies.
- The exact order of implementation of therapies depends on local availability, the side-effect profile of the treatment and the preference of the patient.

The World Health Organization (WHO) 3-step analgesic ladder

The WHO analgesic ladder was developed in the early 1980s to manage cancer pain (Table 17.3). It is successful in controling over 80% of cancer patients who suffer from pain, and has subsequently been adopted for use with all other types of pain. Pain treatment is initiated using the drugs for mild-to-moderate pain listed on the first step, with progression up to step 2 and 3 for severe pain. It utilises conventional analgesic drugs and adjuvant drugs. Adjuvant drugs are predominantly targeted for neuropathic pain, and include drugs such as antidepressants, anticonvulsants and antiarrhythmics.

- **Step 1** – Non-opioid analgesics are derived from three types of compounds: aniline derivatives such as paracetamol, aspirin and other acidic non-steroidal anti-inflammatories (NSAIDs), and non-acidic pyrazole drugs like phenylbutazone and dipyrone.
  - There are over 20 different NSAIDs.
  - When NSAIDs are used for longer than a few weeks, the side-effect profile increases. They are responsible for 20% of hospital admissions for upper gastrointestinal perforation or haemorrhage.

Table 17.3 WHO analgesic ladder	
Step 1	Paracetamol NSAIDs or COX 2 inhibitors
Step 2	Codeine, dihydrocodeine, often prescribed as co-analgesics Co-codamol = **co**mpound of **cod**eine 30 mg/paracet**amol** 500 mg
Step 2 → 3	Tramadol
Step 3	Morphine, diamorphine, pethidine, methadone. Fentanyl, oxycodone. Hydromorphone

Adjuvants	Antidepressants – amitriptyline
	 Anticonvulsants – gabapentin, pregabalin, carbamazepine
	 Antiarrhythmics – lidocaine, mexilitine
	 Miscellaneous – ketamine (NMDA antagonist)
	                        – clonidine (alpha 2 agonist)
	                        – capsaicin

- Aspirin is rarely used as an analgesic because it has a high incidence of the side effects common to NSAIDs.
  - Phenylbutazone, the only pyrazole available in the UK, is restricted for resistant ankylosing spondylitis due to the incidence of aplastic anaemia and agranulocytosis.
- **Step 2** – The use of the less potent opioids such as codeine and dihydrocodeine is commonly practised. These drugs are usually taken in combination with paracetamol.
- **Step 2 to 3** – Tramadol is a drug which has dual mode of activity. Tramadol has been proposed as a drug which bridges the gap between steps 2 and 3.
- **Step 3** – Potent opioids are required for severe acute pain and cancer pain. Morphine is the standard drug, and is usually the first and where rapid onset is required, in severe acute pain, it is usually given by intramuscular or, preferably, by intravenous injection. Several other opioids are available which can be used if morphine produces side effects:
  - oral oxycodone
  - transdermal application of fentanyl or buprenorphine
  - pethidine is rarely used as it has a short duration of action and produces toxic metabolites which can induce convulsions.
- Potent opioids can be used for chronic non-cancer pain conditions but patient assessment at a specialist pain clinic is required.

Adjuvant analgesics

Conventional analgesics used for nociceptive pain are often not effective for neuropathic pain and so adjuvant analgesics are used.

Antidepressants

- The tricyclic antidepressants are the most effective.
- Amitriptyline is the 'golden standard' and is started at a low dose. Analgesic benefit may occur after 2 weeks, but often it requires to be taken for at least 8 weeks before benefits are felt.

Anticonvulsants

- Anticonvulsants have been used successfully for neuropathic pain.
- Gabapentin and pregabalin are modern anticonvulsants which are licenced specifically for neuropathic pain. They are often used as first line amongst the anticonvulsant therapies because they are as effective but have fewer side effects.

Antiarrhythmics

- Lidocaine (lignocaine) and mexilitine block sodium channels and, therefore, can suppress excessive neuronal activity. Lidocaine can only be given intravenously. Oral mexilitine is an alternative.

Topical drugs

- They are not taken systemically and have fewer side effects.
- Capsiacin is a nerve toxin which inactivates the small C pain fibres.
- Lidoderm 5% patch (containing lidocaine) is applied for 12 hours daily.

N-methyl-D-aspartate receptor antagonists

- Ketamine can block the N-methyl-D-aspartate (NMDA) receptor and so reduce allodynia and hyperalgesia.

Regional analgesia

- Regional analgesia comprises the injection of a mixture of pharmacological agents into the painful tissue. The injection can be placed either around an inflamed joint or a nerve.
- Neurolytic blocks (using alcohol, phenol, cryotherapy or radiofrequency) destroy nerves permanently but do not have a permanent effect. The neural system usually regenerates and adapts after 3–6 months and the pain can return or even be worse with permanent sensory and motor deficits.

Physical therapy

Physical therapy includes:

- good foot hygiene
- heat, cold, ultrasound therapy
- braces and splints
- aromatherapy
- local application of treatments such as TENS
- acupuncture – involves the use of very small needles to stimulate certain channels or trigger points. There are various theories for its mode of action, but most evidence indicates that it results in a local tissue response and systemic release of endogenous opioids. Its effects can be antagonised by opioid antagonists.

PSYCHOLOGY

- It is inappropriate to see pain as either physical or psychological; it is always both, as stated in the IASP definition.
- The Gate Control Theory was hypothesised to account for some of the clinical observations made about pain. Such observations include the facts that pain sometimes occurs without apparent cause or does not occur despite

obvious injury (wounded soldier on the battlefield), or persists after tissue healing, or fails to respond to appropriate treatments.

- The pain experience and amount of suffering is dependent on many psychological parameters such as anxiety, past experiences, etc. This applies to acute and chronic pain.
- One of the most commonly used techniques is cognitive behavioural therapy.

SPECIFIC CHRONIC PAIN CONDITIONS OF THE LOWER LIMB

Complex regional pain syndrome

The term 'complex regional pain syndrome' (CRPS) has replaced the terms reflex sympathetic dystrophy and causalgia. CRPS predominantly affects the younger age group with a female predominance of 3 : 1. It is often a mild and transient condition which resolves spontaneously, whilst a small subset becomes chronic and severely disabled.

There are two types of the syndrome:

- CRPS I – symptoms are preceded by tissue injury. It is more common than CRPS II and the incidence is about 1–2% following fracture of a limb.
- CRPS II – as above but occurs after nerve injury and the incidence is around 1–5%.

Both types can be further sub-divided into sympathetically mediated pain (SMP) and sympathetically independent pain (SIP).

Signs and symptoms

- May begin at the time of injury or may be delayed for weeks
- CRPS is manifested by a collection of sensory, vasomotor, sudomotor and motor/trophic disturbances
- Typically the pain is described as constant burning, shooting or aching, and often increases when the limb is dependent
- All patients suffer from hyperalgesia to mechanical stimuli or on joint movement
- Patients can have a sensory deficit of which temperature and proprioception are usually the first to appear and are more common in CRPS II due to the nerve lesion
- The vasomotor effects include colour (vasodilation – red, vasoconstriction/cyanosed – blue or white) and temperature (hot or cold)
- The sudomotor signs include hyper/hypohydrosis and oedema
- Trophic changes present as abnormal hair and nail growth, fibrosis, thin glossy skin and osteoporosis
- Treatments include the general measures described above (WHO ladder and adjuvants) with emphasis on multidisciplinary pain management and restoration of full function. Also sympathectomy blocks can be performed on the lower limb and include lumbar sympathectomy and intravenous regional sympathetic blockade (IVRA).

Finally, remember, there are many reasons why a person should limp. There are even more ways in which to treat it!

Chapter | **18** |

Local anaesthesia

The purification and synthesis of cocaine by Niemann in 1860 led to its subsequent use by Köller for anaesthesia of the eye. The first nerve block was carried out by Halsted in 1884.

Access to local anaesthesia for podiatrists in the UK was first approved by the Chiropodists Board in 1972 and specifically included lidocaine, mepivacaine, bupivacaine and prilocaine.

BASIC CHEMISTRY AND PHARMACOLOGY

- Local anaesthetics are weak bases that are insoluble in water, which are combined with a strong acid to provide a water-soluble salt.
- They have a lipid-soluble hydrophobic aromatic group linked by an intermediate chain (which determines the class of drug) to a charged amine lipophilic group.
- The pKa determines the onset of action. Ionisation of the drug is in reference to the fact that most drugs have a mixture of molecules, some of which are uncharged or un-ionised and some of which have a negative or positive charge and are ionised.
- Amino amides have significant advantages over the amino esters. Amides are basically more stable than esters.
- Lipid solubility is the primary determinant of the local anaesthetic's potency. Higher lipid solubility is accompanied by a greater degree of protein binding, with similar implications for the potency and duration of the anaesthetic's effect.
- Aqueous solubility is another important physiochemical property and is directly related to the extent of ionisation (and, therefore, decreases as pH is raised) and inversely related to its lipid solubility.

Membrane electrophysiology

- Local anaesthetic solutions exert their primary pharmacological action by interfering with the excitation–conduction process of peripheral nerve fibres and endings, thus decreasing the rate and degree of depolarisation of the nerve membrane such that the threshold potential for transmission is not achieved and the nerve ceases to conduct.

- Most of the clinically useful anaesthetic is likely to act by displacement of the calcium (Ca^{2+}) ions from a lipoprotein receptor site on the interior of the nerve cell membrane. This will block the sodium (Na^+) channels. Potassium (K^+) channels are also blockable, but are less sensitive than the Na^+ channels.
- K^+ channels are important in regulating the resting potential. The voltage-sensitive channels can be open, closed or inactivated.
- Local anaesthetics are use- or state-dependent; that is, the degree of block is proportional to the rate of nerve stimulation, i.e. the more rapidly firing neurones are more susceptible than the slower ones.
- Nerve fibres may be of one type or mixed; however, it is generally the smaller C diameter fibres which are more sensitive than larger myelinated A fibres.
- A differential block can be achieved where the smaller pain and autonomic fibres are blocked whilst coarse touch and movement are spared.

CHOICE OF LOCAL ANAESTHETIC AND DOSAGE

- Minor procedures that are quickly completed and which have little post-operative pain can be successfully undertaken with lidocaine.
- If there is a known allergy or sensitivity to a local anaesthetic, then choosing the least chemically similar local anaesthetic is the best decision.
- Longer, and more post-operatively painful, procedures can be best dealt with using a longer-acting anaesthetic, for example bupivacaine or levobupivacaine.
- Whichever agent is chosen it should conform to what are often regarded as the ideal characteristics (Uddin & Reilly 2008) and these are summarised below:
  - complete reversibility (also known as regression time)
  - rapid onset – generally, the quicker the onset the better
  - sufficient and predictable duration – generally in podiatry all the agents provide satisfactory duration
  - low tissue and systemic toxicity
  - distribution/action confined principally to nerve tissue.
- Figures for the maximum safe dose (MSD) are not universally accepted and variation occurs between countries and formularies.
- Generally, UK podiatrists' calculation of MSD is based on body weight, by multiplying the agent in milligrams (mg) by the body weight in kilograms (kg). Table 18.1

Note: generally, the MSD is increased in those solutions which have vasoconstrictors added.

Local anaesthetics used

- Bupivacaine, a very stable hydrochloride and a homologue of mepivacaine and ropivacaine, reported to be four times as potent as lidocaine and mepivacaine. It does have a slow onset time. There is more likelihood of cardiac toxicity with this drug, for example, cardiac arrhythmias and reduced myocardial contractility often resulting in a resistant ventricular fibrillation.
- Levobupivacaine is less toxic than bupivacaine but retains the desirable qualities of being long acting and virtually as potent.

Table 18.1 Commonly used amide local anaesthetics

ANAESTHETIC AGENT

Generic name	Common brand names	Maximum safe dose with plain solution (MSD)
Bupivacaine hydrochloride	Marcain® Sensorcaine®	150 mg (2 mg/kg)
Lidocaine hydrochloride	Xylocaine®	200 mg (3 mg/kg)
Levobupivacaine hydrochloride	Chirocaine®	150 mg (2 mg/kg)
Mepivacaine hydrochloride	Scandonest/Scandocaine®; Carbocaine®	400 mg (6 mg/kg)
Prilocaine hydrochloride	Citanest®	400 mg (6 mg/kg)
Ropivacaine hydrochloride	Naropin®	200 mg (4 mg/kg)
Etidocaine hydrochloride (USA)	Duranest®	300 mg (6 mg/kg)

- Etidocaine is used predominantly in the United States, particularly by the dental profession. It has a rapid onset and medium-to-long duration of approximately 4 hours.
- Lidocaine is one of the most widely used local anaesthetics. It is a fairly fast-acting local anaesthetic, with a variable duration, which may be as long as 3 hours. It is usually used in plain solutions by podiatrists, but from 1998 was available with adrenaline (epinephrine) 1 : 200 000 added as a vasoconstrictor to certificated podiatrists in the UK.
- Lidocaine is also used in topical creams, a cutaneous gel applied to skin, under a dressing for up to 1 hour to facilitate pain-free injections, and this is particularly useful with nervous children.
- Mepivacaine is related to bupivacaine and ropivacaine and is less toxic than lidocaine, particularly on neural tissues. Mepivacaine has a less pronounced vasodilator effect than lidocaine, probably because of its slower clearance. It has a longer duration and quicker onset than lidocaine.
- Prilocaine, with an effectiveness and duration of action only slightly greater than lidocaine or mepivacaine, has a safety profile superior to both due to its rapid clearance. Being a toluidine derivative it may produce methaemoglobinaemia.
- Ropivacaine was created for its long-term efficacy, having about 10% less duration than bupivacaine, but with a much safer profile. It also has a more discreet separation between motor and sensory block.

LOCAL AND SYSTEMIC COMPLICATIONS AND TOXICITY

Local

- Needle breakage
- Intravascular injection may pose a clinical risk.

Systemic

Local anaesthetics are very safe and in the doses used in standard podiatry practice are unlikely to cause problems. However, when larger doses are used, as in podiatric surgery, the risks increase.

All local anaesthetics can cause systemic toxicity, but some, for example, bupivacaine, as mentioned above, have more potential for specific problems, in this case cardiotoxicity.

The following areas are highlighted for particular consideration:

- central nervous system (CNS) – Local anaesthetics have an intrinsic ability to cause irritation to the CNS since they readily cross the blood–brain barrier. They stimulate the cerebral cortex, but will then depress the medulla, particularly the vasomotor and respiratory centres. It is then possible that they may feel nauseous and begin trembling and twitching and possibly convulsing. Drowsiness, leading to unconsciousness may follow and, finally, this could lead respiratory failure.
- the cardiovascular system – Although higher doses are required to cause toxicity than with the CNS, an initial increase in peripheral vascular resistance has been noted. The main effect in very high doses would be depression of the myocardium, systemic hypotension due to a generalised vasodilatation and a decrease in myocardial contractility.
- allergic reaction is extremely rare so far as fatalities are concerned, but it is possible to have a number of non-life-threatening situations, such as an urticarial reaction or difficulty in breathing due to oedema in the laryngeal pathway.
- systemic toxicity is far more likely to occur when the anaesthetic is injected intravenously and in large doses.
- hepatic and renal function – In those patients suffering from any liver disorder, for example cirrhosis or hepatitis, care would be needed.
- pregnancy – Known adverse effects, for example foetal bradycardia, have been documented in the literature, although the caution that applies to mepivacaine, and bupivacaine in particular, during pregnancy refers to data collected in animal teratogenic studies. However, since it is known that these agents cross the placenta, it seems sensible to avoid local anaesthetics in the 1st trimester and, as most foot surgery is elective, the procedure may be delayed until postpartum. In emergency situations this debate may not arise.
- drug interactions have been noted, with local anaesthetic agents inhibiting the action of the hepatic microsomes. Drugs such as the monoamine oxidase inhibitors and the procarbazines will require noting.

LOCAL ANAESTHETICS IN PRACTICE

- Any injectable anaesthetic being used should be confirmed as the agent of choice and have its expiry date and batch number noted.
- A needlestick injury poses the primary risk. Re-sheathing needles constitutes over 50% of needlestick incidents in the UK. Disposing of the whole system into a sharps' container is the best option.
- To administer local anaesthetics successfully it is necessary to consider the anatomy of the area and the site of injection. Note any physical/anatomical barriers, for example scar tissue, various skin lesions, superficial blood vessels and infected areas that might impede the movement of the needle or cause damage to the tissues.

Specific sites

- Local infiltration is the simplest of the techniques and requires the deposition of the anaesthetic around and subcutaneously beneath the lesion. It may be used for a variety of skin lesions, for example warts, basal cell carcinoma and various minor excrescencies, and is ideal where electrocautery, curettage or scalpel excision is to be used.
- The digital block is administered for blocking the hallux and any of the lesser digits. There are a number of variations to this technique with each practitioner favouring their own.
- The 'ray block': this is usually associated with the 1st (Mayo) and 5th rays and is a highly effective technique for anaesthesia of the forefoot, for example for bunion, lesser ray procedures and neuroma.
- More extensive anaesthesia is achieved by blocking the nerves around the ankle. The nerves involved are the posterior tibial, saphenous, sural, deep and superficial peroneal.
- Posterior tibial nerve is the larger of the two branches of the sciatic nerve. At the ankle it runs medially in the neurovascular bundle behind the posterior tibial artery passing behind the medial malleolus and flexor retinaculum, and then giving off calcaneal branches before dividing into the medial and lateral plantar nerves.
- Although unlikely, putting too much local anaesthetic into the bundle could cause a pressure necrosis, since the nerve lies between the tibial and flexor retinaculum. Aspiration avoids intravascular injection. Approximately 5–10 ml of anaesthetic will be required and there may be a time lag before full anaesthesia is achieved.
- The sural nerve, also known as the lateral cutaneous nerve, continues down the posterior calf and runs behind the lateral malleolus with the short saphenous vein. It is a cutaneous nerve supplying the lateral aspect of the foot and the 5th toe.
- Insert the needle lateral to the tendo-achilles and at a right angle to the lateral malleolus. Advance needle to lateral malleolus and then withdraw slightly. Aspirate and inject. It is possible to inject, with a fanning action, about 1 cm above the lateral malleolus, and this tends to take out the small branches, or one can raise a wheal from the Achilles tendon to the lateral malleolus.
- Saphenous nerve is the sensory terminal branch of the femoral nerve and passes down the anteriomedial aspect of the leg and enters the dorsum of the foot about one finger's width from the medial malleolus. Enter the needle between the tendon of the tibialis anterior and the long saphenous vein.
- The superficial peroneal (fibular) nerves are two terminal branches of the common peroneal (fibular) nerve. It becomes cutaneous between the middle and distal thirds of the leg and divides into two branches, medial and lateral. The medial branch supplies the skin of the mediodorsal aspect of the foot, medial aspect of the hallux and adjacent sides of the 2nd, 3rd and 4th toes. The lateral branch supplies the intermediate and lateral skin on the dorsum of the foot, the adjacent sides of the 3rd and 4th toes and the medial aspect of the 5th toe.
- The deep peroneal (fibular) nerve enters the dorsum of the foot between the tendons of tibialis anterior and extensor hallucis longus tendons. It is covered by the superior and inferior retinaculum and runs deep, roughly following the course of the anterior tibial artery. It supplies opposing sides of the hallux and the 2nd toe. Insert the needle between the two tendons and advance until contact with the bone, aspirate and inject. Anaesthesia will be over the superolateral foot.

- *The popliteal block*: The technique is suitable for more extensive, long duration forefoot and midfoot operations and for more involved rearfoot procedures, where general and spinal anaesthesia is best avoided. This technique does mean that the patient is less mobile for some time following the procedure until motor function returns. However, this block allows a long post-operative anaesthesia, which helps with pain management and allows for a painless application of a mid calf or ankle tourniquet.

Chapter | **19** |

Nail surgery

Toenail disorders that are seen most commonly include those of congenital, traumatic, infectious, inflammatory, acquired and neoplastic aetiology.

Ingrown toenail is the most common abnormality of toenails. Ingrowing toenails are a common cause of pain, disability and absence from work and matricectomy is now the most common surgical procedure.

PHENOLISATION

Removal of part or the entire toenail with phenolisation of germinal tissue is associated with high levels of patient satisfaction and very low regrowth rates.

Phenol and alcohol technique is not an invasive procedure. It is carried out with a local sterile field around the foot and using sterile instruments and dressings. Following local anaesthesia, a digital block and pre-surgical scrub to the toe and forefoot, a tourniquet is applied; the tourniquet should be broad and flat, e.g. Esmarch bandage. The time a tourniquet is in place should be kept to a minimum to reduce risk of swelling after it is released. Ideally this should be less than 30 minutes.

NB: Time of application of the tourniquet, time of its release and the return of the blood to the digit after the nail procedure must be noted in the patient's case record.

Total nail avulsion

A narrow spatula or elevator separates the eponychium from the nail plate.

Use steady pressure, insert the elevator below the nail plate, move parallel to the long axis of the toe until there is separation of the nail plate and the nail bed and matrix. The nail plate is removed by locking Mosquito forceps/ haemostat onto the plate half way between the sulcus and the midline of the toe: roll the instrument dorsally towards the midline. A similar procedure will release the other side of the plate and the nail can normally be lifted in one piece.

Partial nail avulsion

A partial nail avulsion removes the involuted section of nail that is causing painful symptoms within the sulcus. A fine spatula is inserted to free the eponychium from the nail plate: aim for as little separation as necessary to limit tracking of liquid phenol. A narrow elevator is inserted below the nail plate to separate it from the nail bed, as with a total avulsion, but being careful to separate only the section of nail to be avulsed. The section of nail plate to be removed is split by a pair of Thwaite's single-bladed nail nippers, a nail chisel or a combination of both. Liquefied phenol is applied; this should be fresh, free from contamination and colourless, and used as a saturated solution – 80% BP or 89% USP. As a general guide phenol is applied for three separate 1-minute applications. Flush the site with alcohol and avoid contaminating the surrounding area. The area is then dried and the tourniquet is removed with the return of arterial blood flow being noted when the colour returns to the digit.

Alternative

Using sodium hydroxide – the nail plate is removed in a similar manner to the phenolisation technique and a pellet of 10% sodium hydroxide is rubbed into the nail bed and the matrix until the capillaries are seen to coagulate. Application of 30 seconds is insufficient but prolonged healing time occurs with a 2-minute application.

It is essential that the patient is given clear verbal and written advice regarding the signs (and symptoms) of immediate post-operative problems.

SURGICAL PROCEDURES

Incisional matricectomy is used in patients whose history or circumstances do not favour phenol ablation.

Winograd procedure

This involves excision of the medial or lateral nail sulcus with its adjacent nail plate, bed and proximal nail root matrix. A linear incision is made, from the free edge of the nail plate to about 5 mm beyond the eponychium, and is then deepened to the bone. A narrow elevator is inserted distally to proximally in order to free and remove the border of the nail plate. A second elliptical incision joins either end of the first incision creating a wedge of tissue. After removal of the wedge, non-absorbable sutures or skin closures are used to approximate the wound edges.

Zadik's procedure

This is the excision of the nail matrix only. The nail plate is removed and a full-thickness flap is created by extending oblique incisions from both corners of the proximal nail fold allowing access to the matrix, which is carefully excised. Regrowth of spicules of nail is common. For closure the eponychial flap is replaced and the lateral incisions sutured.

Frost procedure

The initial incision is the same as that of the Winograd procedure, but with an added incision posteriorly to give an L-shaped tissue flap for better exposure of the nail matrix. Following deep dissection, the nail plate, bed and matrix are then excised. Sutures or skin closures complete the procedure.

Terminal Syme's amputation

Amputation of the distal half of the distal phalanx significantly reduces the rate of recurrence following toenail surgery. An elliptical incision around the entire nail plate and matrix is carried out and then deepened to the bone and, finally, the nail folds are excised. The distal phalanx is cut distal to the insertions of the long tendons and released from the soft-tissue pulp of the toe. The soft tissues are sutured to give good pulp cover of the remaining bone.

AVULSION USING UREA

A solution of 40% urea softens the nail plate while also dissolving the bond between the nail bed and the nail plate. This is used where patients are not suitable for other forms of nail surgery. The area is occluded with adhesive tape and/or a finger cut from a surgical glove. Patient changes dressing and reapplies the urea once or twice per week with the necrotic nail being debrided at regular visits until symptomatic relief is obtained.

TREATMENT OF SUBUNGUAL EXOSTOSIS

This involves a small outgrowth of bone under the nail plate or near its free edge. It occurs singly and unilaterally, usually involving the hallux.

Aetiology

It is the result of either one single traumatic event or, more likely, multiple minor traumas.

Signs and symptoms

It is slow-growing, rarely exceeding 5 mm in diameter, becoming progressively more painful as it increases in size. It is more commonly seen in patients of 20–40 years of age with a female:male ratio of 2 : 1. The epidermis covering the exostosis becomes stretched and thinned with a bright red colour, which blanches with pressure, and it will present a hard resistance upon palpation.

Differential diagnosis

This would include subungual heloma durum and other soft-tissue lesions, e.g glomus tumour, pyogenic granuloma, subungual verruca and inclusion cyst.

Diagnosis

This is by X-ray on a lateral projection with the involved digit isolated.

Management

Short-term management involves protective padding or avulsion of the nail plate. More permanent relief is achieved by surgical excision either using a minimal incision distally (fish mouth) or by an incision at the hyponychium and a raised proximally based flap. In either case, the lesion is removed and its base curetted.

Chapter | **20** |

Diagnostic imaging

INTRODUCTION

Röntgen's (usually written as Roentgen) accidental production of X-rays in 1895 and the first ever X-ray of living human tissue, his wife's hand, served to advance the course of medical investigation and diagnosis, with ensuing benefits for patients. Diagnostic imaging continues to be one of the most dynamically evolving fields of medicine (Yester & White 2006).

IMAGING MODALITIES UTILISING IONISING RADIATION: SAFETY AND LEGISLATION

The current United Kingdom and European Union regulations: Ionising Radiation (Medical Exposure) Regulations 2000 is the statutory instrument and came into force on the 13th May 2000 (Journal of the European Communities 1997). The central tenet of the new regulations is that all medical exposures are fully justified.

IMAGING MODALITIES

X-rays

These provide a considerable amount of information for the assessment of osseous and, in some cases, soft tissues. The plain X-ray remains the most widely used of the imaging modalities.

Magnetic resonance imaging

MRI has minimal complications or contradictions, does not rely on ionising radiation and can provide highly detailed multiplanar images.

In Podiatry, MRI is useful for normal anatomy and for pathologies involving tendons, ligaments and infections, including osteomyelitis. It can also be used to image compartment syndromes and tumours. In addition, it has a high sensitivity and specificity for Morton's neuroma (George et al). MRI is superior to CT scans and ultrasound for all soft tissue and marrow investigations, but the CT scan will be required when examining the bony cortex and for any bone erosion.

Ultrasound

This is based on the use of inaudible, high-frequency, sound waves to produce images. Similar to radar, these sound waves are sent as pulses; in this case they enter the body where some are absorbed and others are reflected back. The pulses are transmitted via a scan head, which has a number of transducers, i.e. piezoelectric crystals, which convert electrical pulses to sound waves.

Ultrasonography may be used to image any of the soft tissues in the foot. It can be used to identify soft-tissue tumours and trauma, for example a torn tendon. One of its major uses for podiatrists is in identifying a Morton's neuroma and perhaps in establishing a differential diagnosis from a bursa, for example.

Computerised tomography

The CT scan offers major advantages over the standard radiograph:

- it produces 3D images of body tissues through all planes.
- the scan may be done as a plain format or in conjunction with a contrast medium, which can be introduced into the patient's body orally, or via a vein.

The CT scans are individual slices or sections of data ranging from 1.5 to 10 mm. A larger number of thin sections will produce better data for diagnosis. The 2-mm sections are probably the most useful for foot and ankle (Oloff-Solomon & Solomon 1988). The digitised images are displayed on a monitor. Advances in software permit 3D surface reconstructions.

The main advantages of the CT scan are:

- its spatial precision
- its excellent contrast and 3D image.

The main disadvantages are:

- the patient is exposed to relatively large doses of ionising radiation
- soft-tissue differentiation is far inferior to MRI.

CT scans are particularly valuable for examining:

- cortical bone (but not the bone matrix)
- periosteal reactions
- calcification of tissues
- osteomyelitis.

Fluoroscopy

This was first used in 1896 and is an X-ray technique, with the same safety considerations as all equipment using ionising radiation. In modern units the X-rays strike a fluorescent plate that is linked to a computer, which sends the data to a monitor where 'real-time' images are displayed. In some podiatric surgery facilities a C Arm fluoroscopy unit is utilised to ascertain the position of pins, screws and possibly joint implants.

Fluoroscopy is also used in a variety of other situations, including endoscopy, imaging of the gastrointestinal tract and in a process called digital subtraction angiography (DSA).

Dual energy X-ray absorptiometry

DEXA is another use of ionising radiation and is used for the evaluation of the bone mass. It more accurately assesses whether the bone is osteoporotic than plain X-rays.

X-ray radiogrammetry

DXR is used to quantifying bone loss, particularly in rheumatoid disease.

Nuclear medicine imaging

NM imaging is not a first-line modality; however, radioactive isotopes are used in a variety of clinical situations where plain radiography may have failed to identify pathology. This method of imaging is useful in the identification of:

- tumours, particularly metastases
- osteomyelitis
- soft-tissues infections
- trauma
- degenerative changes found in neuroarthropathy, particularly in the diabetic foot
- stress fractures.

PLAIN RADIOGRAPHY – COMMON RADIOGRAPHIC PROJECTIONS

"The plain radiograph is still an indispensable tool and should form the cornerstone of imaging protocols. It is quite cheap, enjoys the highest spatial resolution, and is easily reproducible."

(Cassar-Pullicino 2002:58)

A radiographic *projection* refers to the direction that the X-ray beam travels through the body. This term describes a positioning technique and not the radiological image that is created.

Position refers to that part of the body that is closest to the X-ray film. It includes information such as whether the X-ray is taken weight on or off, or a definition of the angle.

There are over 20 different projections of the foot and ankle (Table 20.1), but in daily practice only a small number of these are utilised.

The dorso-plantar projection

D/P (also known as the anterior-posterior view, A/P) is the most frequently used projection for the foot, and one that is best done on weight bearing. The beam is directed 15° cephalically, thus eliminating any distortion caused by the natural

Table 20.1 Projection techniques

	OPTIONS	TECHNIQUE
Dorsoplantar projections	Weight on or off	Vertical or 15° cephalic
Oblique positions	Non-weight bearing	Medial
		Lateral
	Weight bearing	Lateromedial oblique projection
		Mediolateral oblique projection
Lateral positions	Weight on or off	Lateromedial projection
		Mediolateral projection
Individual toe positions	Weight on or off	Lateromedial projection
		Mediolateral projection
		Dorsoplantar projection
		Oblique positions
Sesamoid positioning techniques	Weight on or off	Posteroanterior axial projection
		Anteroposterior axial projection
		Lateromedial tangential projection
Tarsal positioning techniques	Weight off	Dorsoplantar calcaneal axial projection
	Weight off	Plantodorsal calcaneal axial projection
	Weight on	Harris Beath (calcaneal axial view)
	Weight off	Broden
	Weight off	Isherwood
Ankle positioning techniques	Weight on or off	Anteroposterior projection
		Mortise position
		Oblique positions (internal/ external)
		Lateral positions (lateral/medial projections)

declination of the metatarsals. This projection is particularly valuable for demonstrating the phalanges, metatarsals and mid foot.

Lateromedial oblique projection

This is used frequently for podiatric presurgical evaluation. If weight bearing, the tube head is angled at 45° and if non-weight bearing, the foot is angled to 45° and the tube head remains vertical. This projection gives good visualisation of phalanges, metatarsals and sesamoids.

Mediolateral oblique projection

There are a variety of tube angles identified for this position – 45°, 25° and 30°. This is valuable for evaluating the 1st ray and associated structures prior to bunion surgery.

Lateral projections

These may be weight bearing or weight off, but in both cases the tube head is angled at 90° to the foot. This projection is valuable for showing the whole foot in profile, but some superimposition will obscure certain features.

The lateromedial projection

This is particularly good for identifying subungual exostoses. The hallux, or any lesser toe, can be raised above its neighbours.

Sesamoid positioning

The axial projection is most commonly used for isolating and defining the sesamoids. It is possible to take this view weight on or off.

Tarsal and ankle projections

There are a large number of possible techniques for visualising the rear foot and ankle. The most commonly used projections for the ankle are:

- anteroposterior
- lateral
- mortise.

RADIOGRAPHIC CHARTING

This is the process of employing standardised marking and measurement techniques on the X-ray film to enable comparisons and conclusions to be drawn on a number of features. These features will involve the relationships of the osseous structures, and may be used for pre surgical evaluation, or for biomechanical factors, such as the classification of foot type (Street et al 1980). However, the use of charting for biomechanical examination is rather difficult to justify in most situations, since best practice would be not to expose the patient to unnecessary amounts of ionising radiation.

RADIOGRAPHIC ASSESSMENT AND INTERPRETATION

Any radiograph must be read and assessed accurately. There is a logical and sequential method to this process.

The technical quality of the X-ray is assessed for:

- *detail* – are the structural components, i.e. the bones, clearly discernible?
- *contrast* – is there a clear profile of the part being examined?
- *density* – is the radiograph clearly grey or black enough for the image to stand out?
- *quality* – has the radiograph been marred by handling or processing faults.

Whether one examines the foot from proximal to distal or from distal to proximal, is not that important. What is important is that a consistent method is used for the analysis of each radiograph. Each of the major osseous components can be examined in turn, but care will be needed not to confuse normal structures and only through regular examination of radiographs does it become an accurate and reliable process.

Developmental variants: normal and abnormal

While the adult radiograph demands specialised skills for analysis, the paediatric foot presents an even greater challenge. The clinician will require knowledge of the norms for:

- development of the ossification centres
- the timing of their appearance
- the timing of their closures.

The appearance of the primary and secondary ossification centres varies within an accepted age range. Children rarely develop at the same pace; for example, bone development and maturity in girls is normally 2 years ahead of boys. Cartilaginous models of the tarsus are identified from approximately the 7th to 9th week of intrauterine life and, at the same time, ossification is well under way in the metatarsals and phalanges. Between 24 and 28 weeks' intrauterine, the tarsal bones will begin ossifying, with the talus and calcaneus being ossified at birth. By 2 years of age the lateral and medial cuneiforms are discernible, with the intermediate visible by 3, together with the navicular. The process of ossification in the foot is completed with the calcaneal apophysis and the 5th metatarsal head epiphysis; this will occur at the age of, approximately, 13–15 in girls and 14–17 in boys. It is important that the developing ossification centres follow a recognised pattern in terms of their appearance, their size and shape, and in relation to their neighbouring centres (Oloff & Moore 1992). The growth plates at the epiphyses provide for increase in the length of the bone, whilst the apophyses add bulk and form to the bone. The appearance of the primary and secondary ossification centres, and the completion of ossification in the foot is better referenced from detailed anatomical texts, for example Saraffian (1983), as there are variations of timing within the literature (Oloff 1987).

Variation may present in a number of ways. For:

- size, shape or position of a bone
- density and architecture
- extra bones that may be present
- ossicles at various sites
- supernumerary sesamoids, which are sometimes observed under the lesser metatarsal heads
- part of or a whole bone that may be absent.

The radiologist's skill is in determining which of these features is a developmental anomaly and which is pathologic.

Coalitions may develop between two or more bones in the foot. These begin life as fibrous syndesmoses, are most common in the tarsal\bones and may be:

- calcaneonavicular
- talocalcaneal
- talonavicular
- calcaneocuboid
- cubonavicular
- multiple coalitions.

Diagnosis is based on detailed radiographs employing two or more projections. However, while it may be possible to identify some on the X-ray, others will require MRI or CT scans to enable complete and accurate visualisation.

It is possible to identify up to 21 *accessory bones* (ossicles) within the foot. They may be unilateral or bilateral, and are considered as normal variants. They are generally asymptomatic, but occasionally, they will need to be differentially diagnosed from a possible fracture. Those most frequently described are listed below:

- os trigonum is found at the posterior aspect of the talus and has an incidence of between 2.5 and 14%.
- os tibiale externum, often referred to as the accessory navicular, is found adjacent to the proximal part of the tuberosity of the navicular and in association with the tendon of tibialis posterior.
- os peroneum is found in the tendon of peroneus longus. It lies adjacent to the lower border of the cuboid or calcaneocuboid joint. Its incidence is estimated at 9%.
- os vesalianum is situated at the base of the 5th metatarsal and is of importance as it may be confused with an avulsion fracture of the metatarsal base.
- os intermetatarseum is usually found as either a separate ossicle, or a spur between the 1st and 2nd metatarsals.
- os interphalangeus is sometimes found on the inferior surface of the hallux.

Osteochondritis or osteonecrosis

There has been a tendency to conveniently group those pathologic conditions where there is an actual osteonecrosis, and those that are merely normal variations or minor growth disturbances, under the general heading of 'the osteochondroses'.

Osteonecrosis is bone death and is seen as part of the pathological process associated with some of the osteochondroses.

Osteonecrosis can be differentiated as an ischaemic necrosis of bone and may be associated with:

- gout
- systemic lupus erythematosis
- sickle cell disease
- thalassaemias
- trauma
- long-term steroid therapy
- alcohol abuse.

Osteochondroses are only seen in the immature skeleton and they may involve the epiphyses and the apophyses. Some are associated with joints, some with growth disturbance and others with trauma. They have a distinctive radiographic appearance characterised by:

- condensation of the ossification centre
- increased sclerosis
- fragmentation and possible collapse of that portion of bone.

Generally, this is followed by 'healing' and restitution of the normal bone architecture. It is important to realise that most will resolve with no residual problems. However, in some cases, for example Freiberg's, there may be a residual problem with the associated joint(s).

Table 20.2 outlines the main types and features.

Bone tumours

The incidence of neoplasia in the lower limb in general, and the foot in particular, is extremely small, with perhaps some 2–4% of all neoplasms being found in the

Table 20.2 The 'osteochondroses'

NAME	SITE	PATHOLOGY	AGE	RADIOGRAPHIC FEATURES
Sever's disease	Calcaneal apophysis	Probably a normal variation in the secondary ossification centre of the calcaneus	10–14	Sclerosis, fragmentation and increased density of the apophysis
Kohler's disease	Navicular	Extremely rare as a true osteonecrosis, rather a developmental variation	3–7	Sclerosis, fragmentation and bone resorption, followed by repair
Freiberg' disease	Usually the 2nd, sometimes 3rd metatarsal head	A true osteonecrosis, which may result in an osteoarthritic joint in the adult	12–18	Osteonecrosis, flattening of metatarsal head, with subchondral bone fracture, thickening of the cortex and neck of the metatarsal, proximal phalanx may become moulded concavely
Iselin's disease	Base of the 5th metatarsal	Traction apophysitis, with no osteonecrosis	11–15?	There may be fragmentation of the apophysis, but this is accepted as a developmental anomaly
Treve's disease	Affects the sesamoids	A true osteonecrosis	15–20	Irregular sesamoid with fragmentation and a mottled appearance
Buschke's disease	The cuneiforms are affected	Not an osteonecrosis A temporary anomaly of ossification	11–15	Change in the shape of the cuneiform and an increased radiodensity
Blount's disease	Posteriomedial portion of the proximal tibial metaphysis/epiphysis	Not a true osteonecrosis Two forms described originally, infantile and adolescent	1–3 6–13	Medial epiphysis is poorly developed
Osgood-Schlatter's disease	Tibial tuberosity	Not a true osteonecrosis May be associated with trauma, jumping and running sports	11–15	Fragmentation and sclerosis of tibial tubercle
Sinding-Larson-Johansson disease	Patella	Not a true osteonecrosis. Associated with traction/stress	10–14	Osseous fragmentation of lower aspect of patella
Legg-Calve-Perthe's disease	Capital femoral epiphysis	A true osteonecrosis, which may predispose to osteoarthritis in the adult	2–16	Fragmentation and compaction of subchondral bone Fracture of the necrotic bone Flattening and sclerosis of the ossification nucleus. Collapse of femoral head
Osteochondritis dessicans	Talar dome and lateral aspect of medial femoral condyle	Osteonecrosis	12–18	A defined area of subchondral bone circled with a marked radiolucent ring

foot (Helm & Newman 1991). Bone tumours may be benign or malignant, with the malignant varieties representing less than 1% of all tumours (Shaylor et al 2000). Some may arise directly from the bone, or from adjacent non-osseous structures.

The identification of any neoplasm needs the expert eyes of the consultant radiologist, who will usually base the diagnosis on a number of criteria. Plain radiography may not be sufficient and other imaging modalities are likely to be employed to confirm a diagnosis.

The main benign tumours are:

- *aneurysmal bone cyst:* Mainly seen in children and young people from age 5 to 30 years.
- *solitary osteochondroma*: Perhaps more familiar to podiatrists as an osteocartilaginous exostosis.
- *simple (solitary) bone cysts:* These are common in children and are not thought of as neoplastic. Generally, they are not painful and are often discovered by chance.
- *osteoid osteoma*: These form approximately 11% of all benign neoplasia. They are found in long bones, but are recorded within the foot, with a predilection for the talus and calcaneus. Young people from 5 to 25 years are most commonly affected (Shook 2003).
- *giant cell tumour:* An uncommon tumour, particularly in the foot, which, although benign, may be very aggressive locally.
- *enchondroma*: The origin of this benign lesion is cartilaginous. These are more commonly found in the phalanges of the hand, but may present in the foot, rarely are they discovered on the axial skeleton. The age range is between 10 and 35 years of age.
- *chondroblastoma*: This is an uncommon lesion comprised of immature cartilage cells. They are mainly seen in the leg around the knee, but have been reported in the foot, in particular, the talus and calcaneus.

Where considered necessary, the above tumours may be removed by surgery and/or curettage.

The main malignant bone tumours that are found throughout the body, though they are rare in the foot, are:

- *chondrosarcoma*: Like the enchondroma, these have a cartilaginous origin. They tend to affect older adults and are very rare in children. In the foot, they may be seen in any bone, but are more common in the calcaneus and talus.
- *ewing's sarcoma:* One of the most aggressive of all bone tumours, described as a non-matrix-producing round-cell tumour. Its predilection is for the long bones of the leg, and in the foot most commonly in the calcaneus. Mainly affects young people, particularly around the middle teens.
- *osteogenic sarcoma*: This highly malignant neoplasm also has a peak occurrence in younger people, with ages ranging from 12 to 30 years and is more common in males. In the foot, it is mostly found in the calcaneus.

Because of their relative rarity, and the fact that they may be unobserved or misdiagnosed, the treatment of these highly dangerous tumours is sometimes delayed. Imaging and bone biopsies will usually confirm the lesion.

Bones, joints and connective tissues

The arthritides form a complex group of joint and connective tissue diseases, many with a predilection for the foot. In the early stages of these diseases radiology may not be of primary importance, rather, clinical and laboratory investigations may be of more value.

The disorders may be classified on the basis of:

- the underlying pathology
- the radiographic characteristics.

The fundamental radiographic characteristics are represented by either a hypertrophic or an atrophic reaction.

Osteoarthritis

OA represents a hypertrophic reaction. Osteoarthritis is common in the foot, particularly in the 1st metatarsophalangeal joint (MTPJ), the metatarsocuneiform, and the naviculocuneiform and talonavicular joints.

The characteristic features associated with OA are:

- focal destruction of the articular cartilage
- osteophytosis
- metatarsosesamoid involvement
- narrowing of the joint space
- subchondral sclerosis together with cyst formation.

Rheumatoid arthritis

RA is a seropositive, inflammatory polyarthritis with various non-articular manifestations. Its course can be highly variable, as is the prognosis. However, the disease tends to follow a relapsing and remitting course in most sufferers. It is still the most common of the inflammatory arthritides. RA has a tendency to begin as a synovitis in the small joints of the hands and feet. The disease may attack any of the pedal joints, but is generally associated with the MTPJs. Involvement of the mid- and rearfoot joints also occur. Radiographs will usually provide good detail at the MTPJs, but imaging the rearfoot will require several views and possibly different modalities.

The radiographic evidence may show:

- early joint space distension
- inflammation and hypertrophy of the synovium
- effusion into the joint
- joint space narrowing
- periarticular osteopenia and erosion
- secondary osteoarthritic damage
- subluxations and dislocation of one or more joints
- ankylosis of the joint(s).

The spondyloarthropathies

These are a group of seronegative arthritides sharing common features:

- peripheral asymmetrical arthritis
- sacroiliitis, evident on X-ray
- seronegative for rheumatoid factor
- no nodule formation
- associated with HLA B27
- genetic transmission.

Ankylosing spondylitis

This is a chronic inflammatory disorder, mainly affecting the axial skeleton; however, involvement of the peripheral joints is not uncommon. It is most common in young males. Enthesopathy may occur at certain sites:

- the heel
- the spine, leaving scars and new bone formations, known as syndesmophytes, at the junction of the vertebral bodies.

As the condition progresses changes may be discernible on radiograph and the use of a CT scan early in the disease may reveal some evidence of osseous changes, while the use of MRI may reveal specific changes, for example inflammation in the bone marrow adjacent to the joints.

Reiter's disease

This is mainly seen in young males, and is normally associated with a gastrointestinal or sexually transmitted organism, and manifests as a classic syndromic triad of non-specific urethritis, reactive arthritis and conjunctivitis. Foot and lower-limb involvement is high with possible:

- synovitis of the small foot joints
- enthesopathy at the attachment of the plantar fascia and the tendo-achilles
- swollen 'sausage' toes (dactylitis)
- ketatoderma blennorhagia affecting the plantar skin.

Psoriatic arthritis

This is commonly associated with psoriasis, but only approximately 6–8% of psoriasis sufferers actually develop both. Five clinical patterns are observed:

- asymmetrical oligoarthritis – 35%
- symmetrical seronegative arthritis – 30%
- sacroiliitis/spondylitis – 15%
- distal interphalangeal joint arthritis (IPJ) – 15%
- arthritis mutilans – 5%.

Radiological evidence consists of small joint involvement in hands and feet. The IPJ may exhibit marginal erosion of the bone with adjacent areas producing a proliferation of new bone, often referred to as 'whiskering'. Osteolysis may occur in the metatarsals and phalanges resulting in their compaction, sometimes referred to as 'mushrooming' or 'telescoping' of the digits. In the rare, but severe arthritis mutilans, there may be a 'pencil in cup' deformity of the metatarsal. Periostitis and erosion of the terminal phalanges is also common. Ankylosing spondylitis and Reiter's, involvement of the entheses is widespread, with the calcaneus often involved. Differential diagnosis should be established between this and RA, or the spondyloarthropathies.

Systemic lupus erythematosus

This is a connective-tissue disorder with a wide range of joint and other tissue manifestations. It is an autoimmune disease and predominates in females. There will usually be a symmetrical involvement of the wrists, knees and metacarpophalangeal and MP joints, as well as the proximal IPJs in hand and foot.

Systemic sclerosis (scleroderma)

This is a complex spectrum of disorders with wide-ranging involvement of the skin, skeleton and major organs. There may be an arthralgia, but there is little erosion in most cases. The most interesting of the radiological manifestations is subcutaneous calcification and possible resorption of the terminal phalangeal tufts (Black 2002).

Gout

Of the crystal deposition diseases, gout is the most frequently encountered by podiatrists. It represents a group of disorders characterised by a hyperuricaemia leading to the deposition of crystals of monosodium urate monohydrate in the tissues, this in turn leads to an inflammatory reaction. It may attack any joint, but over 70% are seen in the 1st MTPJ.

Radiographic evaluation will not show changes in the early stages of the disease (Nuki 1998). However, if it is chronic and poorly managed 'punched out' erosions may develop at the joint margins. Some subchondral sclerosis may be evident and secondary OA may develop with some osteophytosis. Tophaceous deposits in the soft tissue may show on the X-ray.

Fractures – an overview

"A fracture is dissolution in the continuity of a bone which may be complete or incomplete."

(Gamble & Yale 1976:138)

The plain radiograph will usually be excellent for the identification of most fractures, providing that one or more views are taken from different projections to confirm the diagnosis. However, it is occasionally necessary to use a different imaging modality to confirm the diagnosis where there is difficulty in identifying a suspected fracture. NM scintigrams will often show a 'hot spot' where there may be a stress fracture. CT scans can also disclose difficult-to-see fractures.

There are different types of fracture and they are often described as:

- simple fracture: where there are only two segments of bone
- comminuted fracture: where there will be multiple fracturing of the bone with a number of separate bone segments
- impacted fractures: where one bone has been jammed with great force against another
- open or compound fractures: where the skin is penetrated and the bone exposed through the wound
- complicated fractures: where the deeper structures, together with blood vessels and nerves, are involved
- avulsion fractures: where there is a forceful tearing of soft-tissue structures
- stress or 'overuse' fractures: where a fracture occurs as a result of multiple or repetitive damage, as opposed to a single event
- pathologic fractures: where there is an underlying pathology, for example a neoplasm
- greenstick fractures: generally seen in children and are represented by an incomplete breakage through the bone. The fracture line traverses the cortex incompletely, so that the bone bends rather than snaps.

Chapter | **21** |

Podiatric surgery

PATIENT SELECTION FOR SURGERY

- The basis of patient selection is deciding when to operate and when not by balancing risks against benefits.
- The decision-making process is multifactorial and needs to be based on the patient's physiological, medical, psychological and podiatric status as well as their personal circumstances.
- A patient's medical status needs to be considered carefully and becomes increasingly difficult if there are several problems. Where patients have multiple pathologies affecting different body systems the risk is much harder to quantify.
- Psychological assessment is a difficult area, and most practitioners rely on making an assessment based on their interaction with the patient during the consultation:
  - patients who present with a psychological history may be open and able to discuss and rationalise it.
  - very young and very old patients may show more overt signs of their psychological status.
  - however, some patients appear calm and measured at consultation but develop more overt signs of psychological abnormalities when under the stress of the surgery and during the subsequent stages in follow-up treatments.
- Podiatric status is more straightforward.
- Personal circumstances are important:
  - how quickly will they be able to return to work?
  - patients who live alone without any support from family or friends are not good candidates for day surgery.
  - self-employed manual workers often pose difficulties when they are under pressure to return to work as quickly as possible.
  - incorporating the requirement to be off work for a certain period into the consent form is a good way to protect the practitioner against a claim for damages. Home environment, job, dependants and hobbies need to be included.

PATIENT CONSENT

- As a standard for podiatric surgery it would be best to advise patients regarding the risks of infection, swelling, thrombosis, loss of function/stiffness, recurrence of deformity (where appropriate), delayed healing, non-union and the potential to be worse off after surgery.
- Risks specific to the procedure need also to be communicated to the patient.
- The consent process also needs to prepare the patient for what they should expect from their surgical episode, from their arrival at the hospital/surgery centre to the theatre and then to home.
- They need to have a good idea of what the normal post-operative course is for their procedure and how that might be modified according to their progress.
- Consent needs to be documented and the final consent form signed by the surgeon and the patient.
- Consent should be supplemented with written information for the patient to take away so that they can read it thoroughly.
- Consent by minors (patients under 16 years of age) must be made in conjunction with their parents or guardians.
- The use of written information is of considerable help to the process of gaining informed consent.

SURGICAL TREATMENTS

- Surgical treatment is commonly the excisional arthroplasty or the digital arthrodesis.
- Digital amputation is a useful procedure in the right circumstances.

Lesser metatarsal osteotomies

- A long metatarsal can be shortened or a plantarflexed or displaced metatarsal can be elevated.
- Many metatarsal osteotomies have been described over the years; however, the Weil osteotomy, and variations on this, has overcome many of the pitfalls of previous techniques, allowing for accurate control of the metatarsal position, with good internal fixation and a low incidence of non-union.
- Where a purely dorsiflexory procedure is required, in the case of a plantarflexed metatarsal, a Schwartz osteotomy can be used.
- All metatarsal osteotomies carry the risk of either under- or over-correction and, unfortunately, there is no precise way of determining the degree of correction required preoperatively.

Skin plasties

- The use of skin plasties is widespread in podiatric surgery by removing redundant skin and lengthening the skin as in an overlapping 5th toe.
- Two common techniques for this are the 'V-to-Y' skin plasty and the 'Z' skin plasty. Rotational skin flaps can also be used to help close defects after skin lesion excision. There are several variations on these.

Rearfoot surgery

The scope of rearfoot surgery undertaken by podiatric surgeons in the UK has increased in recent years, but is always going to be in less demand than the forefoot procedures that make up the majority of podiatric procedures.

SUTURES

Materials

- These can be divided into absorbable and non-absorbable, monofilament or braided.
- Monofilaments are smooth, single-stranded sutures, which slide through the tissues easily and provoke less tissue reaction but the knots are less secure.
- Braided sutures are woven fibres and are good for tying knots as they grip well and are more flexible but may produce more tissue reaction.
- Absorbable sutures will break down in contact with body fluids and enzymes after 14 days, but take between 90 to 120 days to absorb fully.
- A small percentage of patients will have some suture reaction especially when absorbable sutures are used to close skin which manifests itself as a small pustule.
- Non-absorbable sutures will maintain strength for much longer but need to be removed at about 10–14 days post operatively or after 3 weeks with incisions on the plantar aspect of the foot.
- Sutures come in a range of sizes and these are expressed in '0's. Most podiatric procedures utilise sutures in the range 2-0 (thick) to 5-0 (thin).
- The needle can be straight or curved and the point can be ground in one of several ways. Curved needles are used most commonly in foot surgery.
- The choice of sutures for different procedures is mainly dependent on preference.

Techniques

- Interrupted sutures comprise a simple loop that is tied off. Usually a row of similar sutures is used or they can be interspersed with other types of stitch such as mattress sutures to give additional strength to a wound.
- Mattress sutures involve an extended loop of suture:
  - horizontal mattress sutures allow a wider loop and a strong everting force on the wound edges
  - vertical mattress sutures also evert the wound well but allow for stronger anchoring of the suture material, which is useful if the structures are under tension.
- Cross-over suture is a double simple suture that allows for fewer individual sutures to be needed to close a wound with the advantages of the simple suture.

Continuous

- Running suture is a continuous suture that allows for speedy closure with knots needed at intervals or at the ends of the wound.
- Continuous locking suture is called blanket stitch in embroidery terms. This is useful as it enables tension to be kept on the loops while you work along a wound.
- Subcuticular is a continuous skin closure. The suture is buried for some or all of the wound length. It can be carried out with either removable

non-absorbable sutures or absorbable sutures. If non-absorbable are used then periodic bridges are placed to allow easier removal of the suture in sections. Steristrips are often used to augment a subcuticular suture to help maintain wound edges together.

TISSUE HANDLING

- The amount of swelling and inflammation post operatively, will always be greater if a procedure is carried out roughly. Thinking physiologically, at a cellular level, will help the surgeon to visualise what is going on and appreciate how every interaction made will affect the foot. Tissue handling should be gentle, taking care not to overstress the wound edges and the structures being retracted.
- Making incisions the right size for the procedure is important; too small, and the wound needs to be stretched too much to gain access; too large, and unnecessary tissue damage occurs. Excessive undermining of the skin and dissection of the layers is likewise best avoided. The more that the inflammatory process is initiated by surgery, the more swelling will occur, placing pressure on the wound and with it subsequent fibrosis that will bind the tissue layers together.
- Atraumatic technique is the term used to describe careful surgical technique and no more damage should be caused than is necessary.
- Incision planning is also important and time spent accurately locating the anatomical landmarks and drawing the incision preoperatively is valuable, ensuring that the incision is correctly located.
- Good tissue handling is rewarded by better outcomes from surgery and patients suffer less pain, less swelling and gain better function.

POST-OPERATIVE DRESSINGS

- The post-operative dressing has the following roles:
  - creating an environment to encourage wound healing
  - forming a barrier to prevent contamination
  - maintaining antisepsis
  - supporting the wound and control of swelling
  - splinting the foot/toes where correction of deformity has been achieved
  - ensuring absorption of blood or tissue fluid
  - being small enough to allow clothes to pass over the foot and for the patient to be able to have some limited mobility
  - the dressing should be non-adherent to allow for a pain-free removal.
- These objectives can be met using a combination of layers. These are:
  - the inner or contact layer is usually a non-stick layer such as Bactigras or Mepitel.
  - the middle layer is commonly plain gauze or a woven-woollen-type bandage such as a Velband or Softban. Several layers are used to allow the pressure applied from the outer layer to be spread evenly. This layer is also the main absorbent layer for fluids.
  - the outer layer is usually an elasticated layer comprising several layers gently stretched to add an even compression over the whole surface of the dressing.

- a surface layer of a compressive stocking type of layer such as Tubigrip, up to just below the knee, can be used to protect the dressing as well as giving compression.
- with certain procedures, it is advisable to use a rigid cast to immobilise and support the foot. Casts can be either non-weight bearing or designed to allow for limited ambulating. The casts for allowing weight bearing need to be stronger to support the forces of weight bearing.

POST-OPERATIVE COMPLICATIONS

Infection

- The incidence of infection in podiatric surgery is quoted at anything from 10% down to less than 1%.
- Many factors affect infection rates and good technique helps to reduce the risk.
- The environment is also very important. Where operating theatres are used by other specialties, the rates of infection are often higher than sole-purpose facilities.
- Aspects of the patient's health may give them a higher infection risk.
- Infection usually becomes apparent from about 5 days post operatively onwards, the commonest symptom of which is pain.
- Management of infection should encompass appropriate antibiosis, lavage of the wound to remove debris and pus, and debridement of necrotic tissue.
- Frequent dressing changes are required along with close monitoring to check for deterioration or improvement of the infection.
- Swelling after foot surgery is to be expected. Physical therapy can help to reduce swelling, but in some patients the swelling does not respond to this and it is simply a case of time to allow the swelling to resolve naturally.
- Post-operative oedema is the commonest problem to be dealt with on a daily basis.
- Dehiscence is where the wound opens post operatively with failure of healing and may be attributable to poor technique with over-aggressive retraction and stress on the wound margins, or infection.

Haematoma

- A haematoma may form from any dead space left. If there is much potential dead space in a wound then the use of a drain will allow bleeding to exit on the surface rather than pool within the foot. Generally, good wound closure with a compressive dressing over the top will go a long way in preventing haematoma formation.
- Joint stiffness – Any sort of joint surgery carries with it the risk of joint stiffness following the procedure.
- Hypertrophic scarring results in raised, enlarged scars. These may be symptomatic, depending on the site. Careful history taking will go a long way in finding out whether individuals are prone to hypertrophic scars.
- Transfer metatarsalgia is a risk with any metatarsal surgery. It is generally a problem when carrying out osteotomies that will, by their very nature, bring about a certain amount of loss of bone and subsequent shortening. Compensating for shortening by using good osteotomy design and appropriate fixation will help to control the amount of shortening and allow for accurate reconstruction.

- Avascular necrosis (AVN) is the death of bone following vascular compromise. This is a particular problem with osteotomies.

Chronic regional pain syndrome

- CRPS is not a common postoperative complication but the incidence may well be higher than realised as some cases evade diagnosis. The warning features of CRPS are pain out of all proportion to what would be expected and that extends well beyond that which would be normal for the type of surgery that has been undertaken – *hyperalgesia*. Patients are generally hypersensitive and will find light touch painful – *allodynia*.

DIGITAL DEFORMITIES

- The majority of toe deformities are acquired and may be secondary to other forefoot problems, such as hallux valgus, or secondary to injuries, such as plantar plate rupture, often leading to a hammered second toe.
- Generalised toe deformities, affecting all or most of the lesser toes, are more likely to be related to biomechanical dysfunction.
- Flexor stabilisation is where the flexor muscles are called in to play to attempt to stabilise an overpronated or unstable/hypermobile foot during the stance phase of gait.
- Flexor substitution occurs where the flexor digitorum longus is functioning to assist the plantar flexors of the foot.
- Extensor substitution exhibits itself in the swing phase of gait. This occurs where the foot is struggling to dorsiflex sufficiently to clear the ground during swing phase.
- The adductovarus or 'curly' toe is usually seen in the 5th toe and to a lesser degree the 4th and then the 3rd toe. The theory for this is that the pull of the flexor digitorum longus (FDL) is from the medial malleolus rather than straight in line with the toe. While the pull of flexor accessories (FA)/ quadratus plantae (QP) is supposed to straighten the pull of the FDL, it is ineffective on occasion.
- Mallet toe deformity is where the flexion deformity occurs at the distal interphalangeal joint (IPJ). This occurs in a long toe or in toes where flexibility at the posterior IP joint is reduced, such as following PIP joint arthrodesis.

HALLUX VALGUS

Procedures

- Simple bunionectomy is indicated where a large medial eminence is causing the patient's symptoms.
- Distal metaphyseal procedures (DMO) are perhaps the most widely used procedures for hallux valgus correction and there are many variations:
  - straight osteotomies, such as the Wilson procedure.
  - angled osteotomies, such as the Austin which offer more stability than the straight osteotomy
  - curved osteotomies
- Fixation techniques also vary and range from multiple screw fixation to K-wires.

- Generally, distal procedures offer a relatively rapid rate of recovery and earlier weight bearing post operatively than more proximal procedures.
- One of the main criticisms of DMOs is the incidence of avascular necrosis.

Mid-shaft procedures include:

- these are a good compromise between basal and distal procedures as they are capable of better degrees of correction than distal procedures but without the need to keep patients non-weight bearing for as long as with basal procedures.
- the most popular mid-shaft procedure is the Scarf osteotomy, which gives a stable osteotomy when adequately fixed and will provide early return to weight-bearing activities, similar to the distal procedures.

Basal procedures include:

- the Lapidus procedure or metatarsocuneiform joint fusion is another alternative. This adds a degree of rearfoot stability by stiffening the medial column and so reduces subtalar joint (STJ) pronation.
- in Hallux procedures it is increasingly common for metatarsal correction to be accompanied by a closing wedge procedure on the proximal phalanx (Akin procedure) (Figs 21.1, 21.2). The rationale is that the hallux needs to be straight, post operatively, for the tendons to be exerting force in a straight line.

Evaluation

- There are many factors to take into account when selecting a procedure or technique which include: the patient's age and levels of activity, the severity of the deformity and the degree of degenerative joint changes present, which will need radiographic assessment.

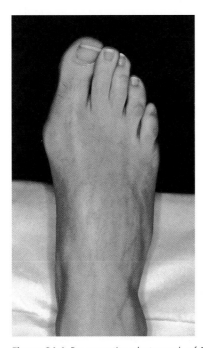

Figure 21.1 Pre-operative photograph of DMO/Akin patient.

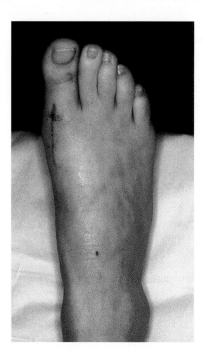

Figure 21.2 Post-operative photograph of the same DMO/Akin patient.

- The intermetatarsal angle has been used to decide if a distal, mid shaft or basal procedure is indicated. The intermetatarsal angle is perhaps of limited value in isolation as it is only one parameter.
- Another method of assessing the amount of displacement necessary is to measure the width of the 1st metatarsal and then the amount of displacement required to move it to its corrected position. This gives a displacement ratio expressed as a percentage of the width of the metatarsal.
- The design of an osteotomy relates to the degree of intrinsic stability. Angled bone cuts giving interlocking fragments are generally more stable than straight osteotomies.
- The manner in which an osteotomy is fixed is also relevant as to how stable it is: the stronger the fixation the greater displacement that can be held adequately.
- The degree of intrinsic stability of an osteotomy will dictate how the patient is managed post operatively.
- Unstable osteotomies usually need to be immobilised with a cast and the patient kept non-weight bearing for a period of time.
- Maintaining a foot non-weight bearing for a period post operatively requires that a patient walks with crutches or uses a wheelchair.
- All of these factors need to be assessed pre operatively; it is not simply a case of looking at the foot or the X-rays as a basis for a decision.

Hallux valgus syndrome

- Hallux valgus is described as being a disorder of the 1st ray, the components of the deformity being metatarsus primus varus and hallux abductus or valgus, and the effects of this spread to other structures and eventually may affect the whole foot.

- The association between hallux valgus and flat foot is not clear. It is possible that the hypermobility in the 1st ray leads to medial instability and subsequent collapse of the foot into a pronated position. Or it could be that the excessive pronation leads to 1st ray dysfunction and subsequent hallux valgus leading to a transfer of load to the 2nd metatarsal.
- The foot pronates and the 1st ray elevates leaving the 2nd metatarsal to compensate with the consequent overloading of the 2nd metatarsal head and a build up of hyperkeratosis over the area and capsulitis of the joint.
- This latter can progress to chronic fatigue in the capsule leading to weakening of the capsule or plantar plate rupture leading to elevation of the 2nd toe and formation of a hammer toe deformity.
- This is further progressed by the hallux moving laterally and exerting pressure against the 2nd toe.
- The hammer toe adds to the problems that the patient is experiencing. Footwear becomes more difficult.
- The patient may be walking on the lateral side of their foot to avoid the painful 1st and 2nd rays in turn leading to pain on the lateral side of the foot and often-associated strain within the leg muscles.
- The midtarsus joint complex may also be starting to show early signs of degeneration due to the changes taking place in the forefoot and the overpronation in the rearfoot.
- Control of the pronation with orthoses may give some relief, although it is rare.
- Correction of the hallux valgus surgically is often a good starting point, accompanied by correction of the hammer toe and also possibly a metatarsal osteotomy to relieve the transfer metatarsalgia.

MORTON'S NEUROMA

- Treatment comprises insole therapy, steroid injections or surgical excision.
- The choice for excision is in where to place the incision.
- A dorsal approach avoids the problem of plantar scarring.
- A plantar incision is more direct and places the incision directly over the nerve.
- The plantar incision requires that the foot remain non-weight bearing for 3 weeks to allow healing to progress and helps to avoid the problem of recurrence or stump neuroma formation.

HALLUX RIGIDUS

- Surgical treatment in early stages is a choice between a simple cheilectomy, where the dorsal osteophytic lipping is resected, through to a metatarsal decompression osteotomy or a proximal phalangeal osteotomy.
- The choices are an arthrodesis, a joint replacement implant or a Keller procedure.

SESAMOID PROBLEMS

- An enlarged sesamoid may give rise to a localised hyperkeratotic lesion. The sesamoid may be enlarged secondary to being bipartite or tripartite, as a result of trauma or degenerative changes. The medial sesamoid is the most commonly affected.

- Evaluation of the sesamoid position can be made radiographically, from an anteroposterior view and an axial or sesamoid view.
- The options for surgical treatment of sesamoid problems are to remove a part, or the whole, of the sesamoid, or to reposition it into a better anatomical position. This latter option would be chosen where the sesamoid symptoms are part of a wider hallux valgus symptom complex.
- Partial removal of a sesamoid, or a sesamoid planing procedure, involves taking off approximately one-third to one-half of the sesamoid, cutting the plantar aspect off the sesamoid in a plane parallel to the weight-bearing surface.
- Removing too much increases the risk of the remaining bone of the sesamoid fracturing.

Chapter 22

Principles of infection control

Prevention of all treatment-associated infection, both in patients and staff themselves, is an integral part of the professional responsibilities of podiatrists.

INFECTION

Terminology

Pathogen

- Pathogenicity – ability of a microorganism to invade a host and cause disease.
- While only true (virulent) pathogens cause infection in a completely healthy host, others can cause infection if the body is weakened in some way.
- These opportunistic pathogens demonstrate that infection is but one outcome of a complex relationship between the body and microorganisms.
- Infection occurs when the balance of circumstances favours a potential pathogen. Given appropriate circumstances, virtually all microorganisms are potential pathogens.

Infection

- Infection is the multiplication of microorganisms in or on body tissues, with an accompanying response by the body's immune system.
- Products of this immune response, for example antibodies against the organism, can be used to detect/diagnose infection or to monitor progress of an infection.
- Contamination merely implies presence of microorganisms which may or may not become established.

Infective dose

- Number of cells/particles of a microorganism required to establish infection – termed the infective dose.

- Pathogens differ in infective dose, some requiring smaller numbers for successful invasion than others.
- For any infectious agent, the greater the number contacting the body, the more probable it is that infection will become established.
- Practical measures taken to reduce the number of microorganisms reaching the patient's tissue reduces the likelihood of infection.

It is impossible to achieve complete absence of microorganisms in the proximity of a patient. However, appropriate cleaning or disinfection will reduce the probability of microorganisms reaching the body in sufficient numbers to cause infection.

The use of sterile instruments and aseptic techniques, to minimise the numbers of microorganisms entering tissue, is required where there is reduced immunity.

Colonisation

Colonisation is when an organism becomes established in or on the body but neither symptoms nor a significant immune response occur. However, colonisation may progress to infection should circumstances subsequently favour the microorganism.

Carriers

Carriers are people colonised or subclinically infected with a pathogen who show no clear symptoms but who are nevertheless infectious.

Sources of infection

A source is a site where potential pathogens grow and multiply. A similar but more variable term is reservoir of infection.

Vehicles of infection

- Many movable objects can become contaminated transferring microorganisms to a susceptible person or body site.
- Some vehicles are naturally mobile because of their lightness, e.g. minute skin scales or respiratory droplets, others are deliberately moved, e.g. instruments.
- Vehicles of infection are capable of transmitting an infective dose but not usually of supporting microbial growth, viruses, in particular, cannot multiply outside host cells, but transmission can occur via contaminated instruments, for example wart viruses, HBV, HCV and HIV.
- It is relatively straightforward to identify high-risk vehicles (for example instruments) and to render them safe by appropriate techniques; individual sources of infection are less easily identified.

Cross-infection

This term is used specifically in clinical contexts to describe the spread of infections to patients from staff or other patients.

Cross-infection is a significant risk to patients and many control procedures are aimed at its prevention.

Portals of entry

- Sites by which microorganisms gain access to the body
- Most pathogens have one usual portal, although some are more versatile

- The respiratory, gastrointestinal and genitourinary tracts are common portals of entry, but microorganisms rarely penetrate intact healthy skin.

Portals of exit

- Sites from which pathogens exit the body and from where they are spread to other people, or other sites on the same body.
- Portals of entry and exit are often one and the same.

Normal flora of the body

Every human body is colonised by a large number of commensal microorganisms – the normal indigenous microflora of the body. Many species, mainly but not exclusively bacterial, occur among the flora, and different body sites support mixed populations of organisms suited to the particular conditions. The skin, mouth, upper respiratory tract and the large intestine are important sites of body flora.

For more information see
Neale's Disorders of the Foot 8E   *page 553*

CHIEF SOURCES AND RESERVOIRS OF INFECTION

The chief sources of infection may be categorised as:

- endogenous – sites of flora or infection in/on a person's own body
- exogenous – infected or colonised people; infected or colonised animals; environmental sources.

Endogenous sources

Infections of wounds and damaged skin are most commonly caused by organisms from the patient's own body which gain access to vulnerable areas on the foot. Examples include:

- *staphylococcus aureus* from nasal flora or, in some people, from colonised skin sites; this organism is commonly involved in external wound infections
- *streptococcus pyogenes* from the throat or mouth
- *corynebacterium minutissimum* from skin flora
- *candida albicans*, a fungal opportunist, for example from skin or mouth
- various intestinal bacteria, including *Escherichia coli, Pseudomonas aeruginosa, Klebsiella* spp., *Proteus* spp., *Clostridium perfringens*.

Exogenous sources

Infected or colonised people

Important and obvious sources of cross-infection are staff or patients with clinical infections of the skin or other accessible sites, for example the respiratory tract. However, human sources of pathogens, including *S. aureus* bacteria, hepatitis viruses or HIV, and fungi, such as *Candida albicans*, are often in symptomless states.

Commoner sources of cross-infection are sites of flora on staff or other patients which, while harmlessly colonising those people, can cause infection if transferred to vulnerable foot tissue, for example approximately 30% of patients and staff will be nasal and/or skin carriers of S. aureus.

Infected or colonised animals

Animals can be colonised or infected by microorganisms which cause human infections. Patients attending for treatment may have been infected from domestic animals, for example by zoophilic dermatophytes such as *Microsporum canis*. Infestation of premises by mice, cockroaches or 'Pharoah' ants may occur.

Such vermin and pests can harbour pathogens, including species acquired from clinical and human waste.

Environmental sources and reservoirs

Survival or growth of microorganisms outside the body is determined by their requirements and the environmental conditions.

All organisms need moisture for growth. Wet sites in clinical areas are, therefore, potential sources or reservoirs. Sites such as soap receptacles, leaks or spillages from pipes or equipment, and residual water in stored utensils, are potential risks. Even aqueous solutions of chemicals, including disinfectants, especially if over-diluted or aged, will allow survival and even growth of microorganisms.

TRANSMISSION OF INFECTION

For infection to occur, microorganisms from an exogenous or endogenous source must be transmitted by some means to a new host or host site.

Direct transmission

- Involves direct physical contact with, or close proximity to, a human source or reservoir
- Staff involvement in direct contact transmission, especially via hands, is of major importance in clinically acquired infections
- This category includes endogenous infection involving transmission from own-body sites, for example wound infections caused by organisms from skin or other sites spread via hands or clothing
- Measures to prevent direct transmission in clinical situations include hand/skin cleaning and disinfection, protective clothing and 'no-touch' techniques.

Indirect transmission routes

These usually involve intermediate vehicles of infection which transfer microorganisms from an animate (including human) or inanimate source or reservoir to a vulnerable host site. A source or reservoir is not directly involved or in close proximity and could in fact be very distant.

Transmission by clinical items

Any contaminated article coming into close proximity or contact with vulnerable tissue is capable of transmitting infection.

Airborne transmission

True airborne transmission, commonly associated with respiratory infections, should have little significance in podiatric procedures.

However, clinic dust is a reservoir of infection and may contain remnants of skin, nail, blood, pus and lesion exudates. Various activities may render it airborne, and thus able to settle afterwards on exposed surfaces. Dry sweeping of skin and nail debris, vigorous movement of curtain screens, overcrowding and unnecessary human activity all increase airborne contamination. While this risk is difficult to quantify, these activities are undesirable near clinical procedures or unprotected sterile items.

Transmission by animals

Vermin and insects may shed contaminants when feeding or defaecating. They may also act simply as vehicles, transferring contamination on their body surfaces from dirty areas, such as drains and disposed wastes.

Faecal transmission

Faecal–oral transmission is of major importance in food- and water-borne infections. While this has no direct relevance to podiatry, note that hands and skin are often contaminated with faecal organisms, including potential wound pathogens, after toilet use, and dispersion of such contamination is more likely if diarrhoea is present.

HEPATITIS B VIRUS (HBV), HEPATITIS C VIRUS (HCV) AND HUMAN IMMUNODEFICIENCY VIRUS (HIV) INFECTIONS

Hepatitis B and hepatitis C viruses (HBV and HCV)

HBV and HCV are two important types of the several viruses which can cause hepatitis, that is inflammation and necrosis of liver tissue. See main text for more information.

For more information see
Neale's Disorders of the Foot 8E *page 555*

HIV and AIDS

HIV (human immunodeficiency virus) causes AIDS (acquired immunodeficiency syndrome), which is the final stage of this virus's progressive attack on the human immune system.

There are currently tens of millions of people at various stages of HIV infection from initial seroconversion to fully developed AIDS. Thus the likelihood of podiatrists unknowingly encountering infected people among their patients has increased greatly.

Implications for podiatrists

- HBV, HCV and HIV are blood-borne but are also present in other body fluids, including semen and vaginal secretions – hence their association with entry of blood through mucous membranes or damaged skin, sexual transmission and mother-to-baby transfer.
- In the podiatry context it is much more relevant that these infections are *not* confined to such high-risk-activity groups and have become much more widespread in the general population. Workers in situations where blood spillage or transfer is likely are at increased risk – for example, health care, prison personnel and police, or other emergency services. Patients who received blood transfusions or blood products before detection or preventative measures were available may also have become infected. Even children, seemingly unlikely risks among podiatry patients, may have been infected by maternal transmission. The crucial point is that a podiatrist will not know whether or not a patient belongs to a high-risk-activity group and the incidence of these infections is now much more widespread among people not in these categories.
- Practitioners must treat all invasive procedures, contacts with blood/tissue fluids, and blood/tissue fluid contamination of instruments as dangerous, however unlikely it seems that the patient constitutes a risk.
- In effect, procedures must prevent transmission from any patient in case they are a source while also protecting each patient from becoming a victim of clinically transmitted infection. All sharps used in procedures must be sterile with particular care in decontamination of re-usable instruments if employed.
- In no way does staff vaccination reduce the necessity for other control measures, which are essential to protect patients from these and other infections.

VARIANT CREUTZFELDT–JACOB DISEASE

Human cases of a new variant of CJD (Creutzfeldt–Jakob disease) appeared and it is accepted that foodborne transmission from cattle to humans occurred.

Although the disease was originally foodborne, the danger now is that transmission via blood or tissue can occur, hence the relevance to clinical contexts. The agent is a prion protein (not a living organism as such) which is highly resistant and it is essential that tissue traces are removed from re-usable instruments by scrupulous cleaning prior to heat sterilisation to avoid its possible survival of the process. Arrival of this new threat is another reason to move towards the ideal of single-use sharps for invasive procedures wherever feasible.

INFECTION CONTROL

The term infection control reflects the realistic objective of reducing infection to the practicable minimum, rather than claiming the ideal of total prevention.

Infection control in clinics must encompass measures to prevent patient infections from both endogenous and exogenous sources, and also to protect staff from becoming infected from patients.

As time progresses higher standards of infection control are expected of professionals, particularly as awareness levels have increased of threats from bloodborne pathogens and antibiotic-multiresistant bacteria, such as MRSA (meticillin-resistant *Staphylococcus aureus*).

The Society of Chiropodists and Podiatrists in the UK has indicated to its members recommended procedures for particular aspects of routine practice.

Terminology

Sterilisation

This is a process which renders an item free from all living microorganisms, that is it becomes sterile (BS 5283 1986). There are no degrees of sterilisation; all microorganisms, including bacterial spores, must be killed or removed. Any process which does not achieve this is a disinfection and not a sterilisation process. Sterilants are chemical agents capable of sterilising, but few can achieve this in routine podiatric circumstances.

Disinfection

A process by which microorganisms are reduced to a level that is harmless to health. In contrast to sterilisation, there are degrees of disinfection; the level of microbial reduction considered necessary being dependent on the item to be disinfected and the infection risk it presents in that situation. Bacterial spores are often little affected. Disinfection, unlike sterilisation, can be applied to living tissue, for example skin, as well as to inanimate articles.

Antisepsis

The destruction or inhibition of microorganisms on living tissues having the effect of limiting or preventing the harmful results of infection (BS 5283 1986).

Antiseptics are chemical agents used to achieve antisepsis; they are usually unsuitable for general use on inanimate articles, for reasons of either lower anti-microbial action or cost-effectiveness.

Some antiseptics inhibit rather than kill microorganisms, this capability being described using terms such as bacteriostatic or fungistatic.

Asepsis

An absence of contamination or, perhaps more realistically, absence of infection (sepsis) resulting from contamination. This should be the objective underlying all clinical procedures. Aseptic techniques are safe methods of working on patients by which contamination is minimised and thus infection prevented – in this context, largely by the prevention of cross-infection and the protection from contamination of damaged foot tissue. As appropriate, both sterilisation and disinfection are employed to achieve asepsis.

Strategies and methods of control

As microorganisms may be transmitted by so many routes, a similarly wide range of measures must be employed in infection control.

All individual control measures stem from three basic strategies of infection control:

1. Elimination of sources and reservoirs of infection
2. Disruption of transmission routes
3. Increasing or restoring host resistance to infection.

Elimination of sources and reservoirs

- Important sources of infection are patients with existing clinical infections, for example septic lesions, fungal infections or verrucae. Successful treatment not only benefits that patient but also eliminates him/her as a source of cross-infection. During a course of treatment, dressings minimise exit of pathogens from such sources. Endogenous infected sites must be covered by dressings before invasive techniques or exposing nearby tissue.
- Podiatrists with clinical infections are clearly a risk to patients.
- Particularly relevant are infections on the hands or other exposed areas of skin, for example furuncles, infected cuts or paronychia.
- Covering small lesions by waterproof plasters and wearing gloves reduces risk to patients, but such measures may not suffice to eliminate the risk, especially in procedures where glove puncture is possible.
- Where there is any doubt, direct contact with patients should be avoided until the infection is resolved.
- Accumulations of dirt or dust anywhere in the clinical environment are reservoirs of infection eliminated by cleaning, with additional disinfection if necessary.
- Clinical waste must not be allowed to contaminate the area and should be disposed of hygienically.
- Collection of patient debris at source is a sensible measure, for example by using a disposal bag underneath the foot or similar measures.
- Wet sites resulting from faulty equipment or plumbing can be eliminated by repair or replacement.

Disruption of transmission routes

Essentially this is achieved by effective decontamination of inanimate vehicles and by procedures designed to exclude contamination at the point of patient contact, the latter including hand/skin disinfection and other aspects of aseptic technique:

- decontamination of inanimate articles is based on cleaning, disinfection and sterilisation.
- cleaning is usually adequate for most general items, such as furniture, utensils and laundry.
- disinfection is necessary when a specific infection risk is known to exist, for example articles in the vicinity of treatment procedures, blood spillages, and for articles which are unsuited to sterilisation but require more thorough decontamination than cleaning.
- sterilisation is necessary for all items penetrating the body or contacting exposed tissues.

See main text for more information of each area.

For more information see
Neale's Disorders of the Foot 8E *page 557*

Hands of staff and skin of patients both require adequate decontamination, the degree necessary being dictated by the circumstances. Whatever method is used, effectiveness depends largely on the care and thoroughness of the operator.

Hands

Handwashing facilities vary, but taps operated without hand contact (for example foot operated) are best, and if ordinary taps are fitted they should be turned off using a paper towel:

- main purpose of routine handwashing is to remove transients acquired from previous contacts, particularly patients.
- although loosely adhering transients can be removed by washing with ordinary soaps, detergent/disinfectant preparations containing chlorhexidine, povidone-iodine or Triclosan are more effective, and on repeated use they also progressively reduce the more accessible flora.
- further reduction of skin contamination is required for some procedures, for example nail surgery.
- note that hand disinfection is not an alternative but an addition to wearing gloves for aseptic procedures.
- hand cream may be employed to offset the drying effects of disinfectant products, but it should be one which is compatible, as commercial products often inhibit disinfection; pharmacists can advise on suitable products.
- recently there has been debate and discussion regarding the use of clinical dress which has sleeves reaching the wrist (DoH Publication 285129 2008). It is considered that the material is a possible vehicle for transporting flora. At this stage there are not any national guidelines formulated but some NHS Trusts in the UK are implementing the wearing of clinical clothing such as "scrub suites" for all clinical procedures. This facilitates hand washing extending to the elbows.

Patients' skin

- Intact skin should be cleaned before disinfection if possible.
- As immediate, effective disinfection is required, alcoholic skin disinfectants are the agents of choice.
- Chlorhexidine is less likely to cause any reaction, although povidone-iodine has wider antimicrobial action; normally either is suitable.
- Friction is an important factor in skin disinfection; rubbing the site thoroughly with the agent (subject to patient comfort) is more effective than merely wiping or spraying.
- Combined detergents/disinfectants (for example Savlon) may be used for damaged skin which requires cleaning. Injections (for example local anaesthetic) present little danger of infection but skin is often prepared by swabbing with alcohol.

Sterilisation

Of the many methods of sterilisation available, only steam at increased pressure and dry heat are likely to be used directly by the podiatrist.

Steam at increased pressure

- Generally recommended for use on clinical materials whenever possible
- Steam hot enough to sterilise necessitates pressure vessels, termed sterilisers or autoclaves
- Saturated steam sterilises articles it contacts, the time required depending on the temperature. Minimum treatments required are:
  - 15 min at 121°C
  - 10 min at 126°C
  - 3 min at 134°C
- Basic types affordable by many practitioners rely on simple displacement of air by steam generated within the steriliser. Removal of air, steam

penetration and subsequent drying are therefore not as efficient in these models. However, these small sterilisers are suitable for rapid sterilisation of instruments, either unwrapped or in steam-permeable containers

- When removed, instruments must be covered immediately to prevent contamination
- A sterile cloth may be used or a lid sterilised separately in the same cycle could be clipped onto the instrument tray.

Where practicable, central sterile supplies units or similar local services should be used as a first-choice option, as these facilities should be able to guarantee sterility of products and incorporate a total quality-management system. See main text for more detailed information on sterilisation.

For more information see
Neale's Disorders of the Foot 8E *page 561*

Protective clothing

- Any serious attempt at aseptic technique precludes contact of the practitioner's bare hands with damaged skin or exposed tissue, that is 'no-touch' techniques should be used.
- Routine wearing of sterile single-use gloves for such procedures should be adopted.
- Apart from patient protection, there is the risk of contamination of podiatrists' skin by HBV, HCV or HIV, and gloves should always be worn after a suitable and sufficient risk assessment for giving injections, changing dressings, cleaning wounds and for any invasive procedure.
- Cuts or abrasions on the hands should be covered by waterproof plasters even when gloves are worn.
- Hands require washing after a gloved procedure as not all gloves are structurally perfect.
- The wearing of masks is unnecessary for minor procedures, including routine dressing changes.
- Situations requiring masks include nail drilling for the podiatrist's protection and nail surgery, where effective masks to filter/deflect organisms from the mouth away from the operation site are necessary.
- Masks must be discarded after each use and not worn around the neck to be donned at intervals.
- Note that drilling of mycotic nails is unwise; not all debris is removed by the drill vacuum and significant amounts escape to contaminate the clinical environment and the practitioner.
- The usual clinical coat is satisfactory for many procedures but needs protection when significant debris is expected.
- A gown, plastic apron or adequately sized impermeable paper sheet or drape would serve the purpose.
- Purpose-made gowns or suits of appropriate material should be used for surgical procedures, and hair should be completely covered by a surgical cap.
- If surgical footwear is fitted, avoid contamination of previously disinfected hands.

Aseptic technique

- Initial disinfection of the patient's skin should be followed by the use of sterile instruments whenever skin is penetrated, accidental breach is likely or previously wounded tissue is being treated.

- Other materials used on or near such vulnerable areas, for example dressings, must also be sterile.
- Single-use sachets of antiseptics, etc., are preferable but, if communal ones are used, individual quantities should be dispensed without contaminating the remainder.

Sterile fields

- A sterile field is an area in which contamination is kept to an absolute minimum, although it is unlikely to be sterile in the full microbiological sense.
- Such a field may be established by starting with a sterile surface and thereafter taking every care to avoid contamination of that area.
- The surface must not be touched by bare hands, and any necessary items are transferred aseptically onto it.
- The initial surface may be formed by a sterile drape/towel, or the unfolded inner (sterile) wrapping of a dressing pack, placed on a disinfected trolley top.
- If pack wrapping is used it must be unfolded by the corners, taking care not to reach over the contents as they are uncovered because contaminants are shed from skin and clothing. Additional items may be slid gently from their sterile wrapping onto the sterile field, or transferred by sterile forceps.
- Outer wrappings are always contaminated and should not be opened near the sterile field.
- Sterile instruments should be arranged in the field conveniently within reach. After use (that is when they are contaminated), they should be placed elsewhere for disposal, or on a separate secondary field (for example clearly to one side) for possible re-use, but not back among sterile items.
- It may prove convenient to use a sterile, empty steriliser tray as a secondary field which can be used later to transport used instruments.
- Contaminated disposable items, for example swabs, should be disposed of immediately and should not re-enter the sterile field. Overall, there should be a one-way movement from sterility to patient to disposal or secondary field.

Waste disposal

- Clinical waste should be placed carefully in bags and sealed before removal to prevent contamination of the area.
- Bags should be colour-coded.
- There is no universal code, though yellow is used in the UK to denote contaminated waste for incineration.
- Bags should not be overfilled and must be removed from the clinical area frequently; at least daily.
- Bags should be stored safely and protected from damage, until removed by disposal personnel.
- Re-usable instruments should be bagged or containerised for return to a central sterile supplies unit, or cleaned before return, or cleaned and re-sterilised in-house, depending on individual arrangements.
- Disposal of sharps requires great care to protect the practitioner and others from the risk of HBV, HCV and HIV infection.
- Sharps must be discarded into a rigid container meeting approved specifications for example BS 7320 (1997), and sent for incineration.

Chapter | **23** |

Medical emergencies in podiatry

Medical emergencies in the daily practice of podiatry are likely to be rare, but some predictable and unpredictable medical events may occur during clinical procedures. Prevention and avoidance can be achieved through the use of careful clinical assessment to identify the 'at-risk' individuals:

- predictable events:
  - cardiac disease
  - diabetic glycaemic control
- unpredictable events range from simple and recoverable situations:
  - vasovagal faints
  - arrest
  - local anaesthetic (LA) toxicity.

CLINICAL ASSESSMENT

- Podiatric consultation must focus on an holistic view of the patient's general health
- Medical conditions and pharmacological history ascertained
- Pharmacological treatments recorded
- Poorly controlled systemic disease results in poor wound healing, infection and bleeding problems.

Significant medical conditions and important symptoms to exclude before commencing treatment are shown below. Table 23.1

CLINICAL MONITORING

- Clinical monitoring should be instigated before, during and after procedural work.
- Any incision or injection required during the procedure requires a baseline heart rate and blood pressure recording before commencing treatment.

Table 23.1 Important medical conditions and symptoms to check for in the initial consultation

SYSTEM	WORRYING SYMPTOMS
Cardiovascular	
Ischaemic heart disease/myocardial infarction	Chest pain, shortness of breath on exertion
Hypertension	Poor control (diastolic >95, systolic >160)
Dysrhythmias	Slow heart rate (<60 bpm, beta-blocker therapy) Faints, palpitations, shortness of breath
Valve surgery/cardiac stents	Check anticoagulation status
Respiratory	
Asthma	Shortness of breath Chest infection
Chronic obstructive pulmonary disease	Current chest infection, extreme breathlessness
Endocrine	
Diabetes	Poor glucose control Postpone if BM >11
Thyroid disease	Uncontrolled thyroid disease
Hepatic/renal	
Dysfunction or chronic disease	Will affect drug clearance, dosing
Central nervous system	
Stroke/transient ischaemic attack	Check anticoagulant status
Epilepsy	Recent or uncontrolled seizures

- In conscious procedures the best monitor is always the patient themselves.
- The practitioner should continue verbal contact with the patient throughout the procedure.
- Continuous echocardiography monitoring (ECG), for heart rate and rhythm, with non-invasive blood pressure monitoring (NIBP), on a 3–5-min cycle, should be used routinely during procedural work.
- Respiratory disease requires oxygen saturation (SpO_2) finger-probe monitoring.
- Post procedure monitoring measuring static BP at 5–15-min intervals until the patient is fit to leave the recovery area.
- Appropriate monitoring facilitates the detection of cardio-respiratory events including:
  - anaphylaxis
  - accidental intravenous local anaesthetic injection
  - cardiac arrest
  - slow heart rates (during vasovagal syncope)
  - hypoxic changes.

Table 23.2 Baseline monitor references

MONITOR	NORMAL RANGE IN HEALTH
Electrocardiograph	Rhythm: sinus, or sinus arrhythmia Rate: 60–100 bpm
Non-invasive blood pressure	Systolic 80–150 Diastolic 60–90
SpO_2	>95%

- Early detection of these changes will facilitate immediate treatments to prevent spiralling deterioration of the clinical situation. Table 23.2

EMERGENCY DRUGS AND EQUIPMENT

- A possibility for incidental or iatrogenic cardiac arrest exists during procedural work when using LA.
- Basic or advanced cardiopulmonary resuscitation on site is needed.
- An emergency trolley in an accessible location must always be available and:
  - be regularly checked and kept stocked
  - provide immediate airway and IV access devices
  - carry drugs to meet resuscitation protocols
  - contain pipeline or cylinder oxygen (depending on the location of the treatment area)
  - contain atropine and epinephrine (adrenaline)
  - carry a defibrillation machine
  - carry Intralipid™, which should also be kept onsite.

PREDICTABLE EVENTS

Cardiovascular

Angina

The anxiety and stress associated with a procedure or an injection can precipitate angina symptoms:

- should an angina attack occur:
  - suspend all procedural work
  - lie patient in a recumbent position
  - offer oxygen if breathlessness exists
  - use the patient's own GTN or nitrate tablet immediately
  - hospitalise immediately if pain unrelieved by GTN.

Myocardial infarction

- If a heart attack is suspected:
  - give crushed aspirin 300 mg orally
  - call emergency ambulance

- continue electrocardiograph (ECG) and non-invasive blood pressure (NIBP) monitoring until paramedics arrive
- cardiopulmonary resuscitation (CPR) required if cardiovascular collapse occurs
- a period of 6 weeks to 6 months should elapse before any elective procedures following myocardial infarction.

Hypertension

- Anxiety before procedures/during BP assessment transiently elevates BP
- Repeat measurement identifies an artificially elevated reading
- If baseline BP persists above a systolic pressure >160 mmHg or a diastolic >95 mmHg treatment is postponed
- Refer to GP for further assessment and treatment
- Poorly controlled BP increases risk of stroke, cardiac and renal complications.

Dysrhythmia

- Patients susceptible to abnormal heart conduction may develop an altered ECG during a procedure.
- The commonest arrhythmia is atrial fibrillation, which requires anticoagulants.
- Anticoagulation increases bleeding risk during procedural work.
- Aspirin is usually continued, warfarin and clopidogrel are temporarily ceased.
- Liaison with GP is required if a drug is to be suspended.

Heart valves/stents

- Valves and stents require permanent anticoagulation.
- Careful assessment of anticoagulation therapy should occur. Close liaison with hospital specialist or GP is essential.
- Anticoagulation therapy for newer drug-eluting stents is continued for 12 months. Non-essential treatments are postponed during this period.
- Antibiotic cover is required prior to procedure.

Respiratory

Asthma presents with wheeze, cough and shortness of breath

- Chronic illness with periods of flare and control
- Controlled with inhalers. A bronchodilator, salbutamol, opens up the airways, steroid to reduce inflammation
- Oral steroids needed to control symptoms
- Treatment avoided during courses of oral steroids. These drugs reduce wound healing and predispose to infection
- Anxiety and stress precipitate an asthmatic attack
- Monitoring the patient's breathing is the best measure of asthma severity.

Chronic obstructive pulmonary disease

- Chronic obstructive pulmonary disease (COPD) has similar symptoms to asthma
- Productive sputum for at least 3 months of the year – commonly referred to as 'chronic bronchitis'

- Occurs in more elderly patients
- Debilitating shortness of breath. Antibiotic and steroid therapy required
- Treatment avoided during steroid therapy
- If the SpO$_2$ is less than 92% on air – increased risk of developing pulmonary difficulties.

Endocrine

Diabetes

- Hypoglycaemia
  - Untreated will progress to unconsciousness
  - If <5 mmol and patient conscious, administer oral glucose
  - If unconscious, IM glucagon 1 mg is given or IV glucose replacement administered (50 ml boluses of 10% glucose)
  - Patient referred to their primary care physician for review
- Hyperglycaemia
  - Usually caused by infection or dehydration
  - Reduced conscious level or coma with ketotic breath
  - Urine test highly positive for sugar
  - Life-threatening condition – managed in an acute medical unit.

Hepatic/renal

Renal failure

- Renal failure causes cardiovascular changes including hypertension.

Hepatic disease

- Autoimmune, cirrhotic or infective diseases of the liver cause jaundice and systemic upset. In severe cases affects blood clotting and drug metabolism.

Central nervous system

Transient ischaemic attack/stroke

- Patients with known cerebro-vascular disease may collapse during treatment and require basic life support.
- In stable conditions anticoagulation therapy affects the treatment options.
- Aspirin prescribed to prevent emboli can be continued.
- Communication and mobility issues in recovering stroke patients pose problems during therapy.

Epilepsy

This is a disease characterised by minor (petit mal) or major (grand mal) seizures:

- minor fits – Can occur frequently. Provided they do not differ from the patient's normal seizure events they need not affect treatment.
- major fits – Involves loss of consciousness and if this occurs suspend all procedural work. Note the following:
  - environment made safe to protect patient from harm
  - trolley sidebars raised
  - beds reduced to the lowest level to prevent patient falls
  - sharp and hard objects removed from around the patient

- once the seizure has ended, patient placed in the recovery position until conscious
- patient may have an episode of urinary incontinence during the seizure
- patient's airway and mouth should not be instrumented
- routine monitoring and observation during the recovery phase
- if seizure lasts longer than 10 minutes an ambulance should be called. Prolonged seizure activity has a detrimental effect on the brain.

UNPREDICTABLE EVENTS

Vasovagal syncope

Dizziness and collapse have many causes including cardiac, neurogenic and metabolic, but the most common cause in an otherwise healthy individual is the simple faint or 'vasovagal' episode

- Exaggerated reflex response to poor blood flow to the heart
- Commonly occurs after prolonged standing, heat or following a large meal
- Monitoring will show a slowing heart rate sometimes with brief asystole with low blood pressure.

Treatment is supportive:

- lie patient flat
- raise the patient's legs
- put head low between the legs if patient is sitting
- postpone procedure
- ensure the patient is recumbent and distracted before the noxious event if susceptible to stimuli-induced vasovagal events
- refer recurrent or unexpected fainting to the GP.

Cardiac arrest

This is the cessation of mechanical heart function and the culmination of many catastrophic physiological events. It is usually due to an overwhelming injury to the heart itself, it can occur due to:

- heart attack or tamponade
- blood clots
- salt imbalance (low/high potassium)
- shock
- low oxygen (hypoxia)
- collapsed lung (pneumothorax).

Treatment

Knowledge of the cause of the cardiac arrest facilitates appropriate hospital treatment to reverse the initiating pathology; however, in the interim the following should be initiated:

- basic life support (BLS) to keep oxygenated blood going to the heart and brain
- mouth-to-mouth and cardiac massage
- 100% oxygen administration
- adrenaline (epinephrine) given every 3 minutes
- a defibrillator attached to the patient
- ECG trace to see if it is appropriate to administer an electrical pulse to stabilise the heart.

Allergy/anaphylaxis

Allergy

Reactions include:
- an innocuous itch
- skin erythema
- histamine release
- antibody-mediated anaphylactic phenomena.

  Common allergies include:
- drug
- chemical
- latex
- local sensitivity to adhesive in plasters.

Anaphylaxis

- Antibody-mediated process
- Most frequently the reaction is associated with antibiotics, particularly penicillin
- Newer amide-type LA drugs are less likely than the old type of ester LAs to provoke this response
- Allergy to additives within the LA ampoule are often the precipitant
- Careful questioning to previous local anaesthetic exposure may give warning to possible allergy, e.g. during dental or surgical procedures and any unusual difficulties and drugs noted.

  Clinically, anaphylaxis can present immediately with:
- IV injections or be delayed by 10–30 minutes when subcutaneous infiltration is used
- a feeling of 'impending doom' caused by a rapid fall in BP
- difficulty in breathing and wheezing
- loss of consciousness
- cardiac arrest.

Treatment

- Resuscitation
- Adrenaline (epinephrine) given early as a 0.5–1 mg IM injection
- IV steroids and an antihistamine should also be administered
- Airway support in the acute phase
- Supplemental oxygen is essential for airway swelling and obstruction
- Transfer patient to A&E
- Following recovery refer the patient to immunology for identification of the allergen
- The practitioner involved must ensure the assessment takes place and inform the patient and the GP of the result
- Patient may opt to wear a 'medic-alert' bracelet
- Update case-notes to reflect the allergy and severity.

Local anaesthetic toxicity

The action of LAs is to block pain transmission from the surgical area. If the LA reaches high concentrations in the blood stream, deleterious effects on the central nervous and cardiovascular systems follow:

- arrhythmia – altered heart rhythm
- weakens heart contractility – cardiovascular collapse

- blocks higher brain functions – seizures and coma
- tinnitus
- tingling or numbness around the mouth.

Lidocaine, ropivacaine and levobupivacaine are less cardiotoxic than bupivacaine but all can cause fatal reactions. Recent interest has focussed on the use of Intralipid to facilitate resuscitation by sequestering the LA in the lipid.

Toxicity treatment (Table 23.3)

Table 23.3 Local anaesthetic toxicity treatment
Prevent by careful injection and regular aspiration Limit dose of local anaesthetic (LA) to maximum dose by patient weight: lidocaine (plain) (3 mg/kg), bupivacaine (2 mg/kg), ropivacaine (3 mg/kg)
Stop injecting and aspirate if symptoms occur
Give 100% oxygen, establish IV access if not already present
Give fluids and epinephrine in 0.1 mg IV boluses to support circulation
Commence basic life support/advanced life support

Administer Intralipid:
   1 ml/kg up to three boluses. Infuse at 0.25 mg/kg/min
   Maximum dose 8 ml/kg

Prolonged resuscitation (>1 hour) may be required depending on LA used

References

Bennett JA 2000 Dehydration: hazards and benefits. Geriatric Nursing 21(2):84–87.

Black C 2002 Systemic Sclerosis. In: Collected reports on the rheumatic diseases. The Arthritis Research Campaign: England.

Boyd PM, Bogdan RJ 1997 Sports Injuries. In: Lorimer DL, French GJ, West S (eds). Neale's Common Foot Disorders; Diagnosis and Management, 5th edn. Churchill Livingstone: Edinburgh, pp 198–201.

Cassar-Pullicino VN 2002 The place of imaging in rheumatological disorders. In: collected reports on the rheumatic diseases. The Arthritis Research Campaign: England.

Gamble FO, Yale I 1975 Clinical foot roentgenology, 2nd edn. Krieger: New York.

Helm RH, Newman RJ 1991 Primary bone tumours of the foot: experience of the Leeds Bone Tumour Registry. The Foot 1(3):135–138.

Journal of the European Communities 1997 Directive 97/43 Euratom.

Kirby KA 1992 The Medial Heel Skive Technique: improving pronation control in foot orthoses. J Am Podiatr Med Assoc 82:177–188.

Kirby KA 2001 Subtalar joint axis location and rotational equilibrium theory of foot function. J Am Podiatr Med Assoc 91:465.

Nigg BM 2001 The role of impact forces and foot pronation: a new paradigm. Clin J Sports Med 11:2–9.

Nuki G 1998 Gout. Medicine 26:54–59.

Oloff J, Moore SG 1992 Diagnostic imaging of the paediatric patient. In: DeValentine SJ (ed.) Foot and ankle disorders in children. Churchill Livingstone, Inc.: New York.

Oloff Solomon J, Solomon MA 1988 Computerised tomographic scanning of the foot and ankle. Clin Podiatr Med Surg 5(4): 931–944.

Oloff Solomon J 1987 Computerised Radiographic Evaluation of the Pediatric Patient. Clinics in Podiatric Medicine and Surgery 4(1):21-36. WB Saunders: Philadelphia.

Perry J 1992 Gait Analysis: Normal and Pathological Function. Slack Inc.: New Jersey.

Saraffian SK 1983 Anatomy of the foot and ankle. Lippincott: Philadelphia.

Schauwecker DS 1992 The scintigraphic diagnosis of osteomyelitis. Am J Roentgenology 158:9–18.

Shaylor PJ, Abudu A, Grimer RJ, Carter SR, Tillman RM 2000 Management and outcome of the surgical treatment of primary malignant tumours of the foot. The Foot 10(3): 157–163.

Shook JE, Osher LS, Christman RA 2003 Bone tumours and tumour like lesions. In: Christman RA (ed.) Foot and ankle radiology. Churchill-Livingstone: St Louis.

Street MW, Johnston KA, DeWitz MA 1980 Radiographic measurements of the normal adult foot. Foot and Ankle International 15:661.

Uddin A, Reilly I 2008 Ropivacaine and levobupivacaine: potential uses in podiatric medicine and surgery. Podiatry Now 11(4):22–28.

Wakimoto P, Block G 2001 Dietary intake, dietary patterns, and changes with age: an epidemiological perspective. Journal of Gerontology A – Biological Science and Medical Science 56:65–80.

Wilson M-MG, Morley JE 2003 Impaired cognitive function and mental performance in mild dehydration. European Journal of Clinical Nutrition 57:S24–S29. Health Source: Nursing/Academic Edition, EBSCO*host* (accessed December 6, 2009).

Yester M, White SL 2006 Advances in medical physics. In: Wolbarst AB, Zamenhof RG, Hendee WR (eds). Medical Physics Publishing. Lippincott Williams & Wilkins Inc.: Philidelphia.

Index